Dr Liam Farrell is from Rostrevor, Co Down, Ireland. He is a former family doctor in Crossmaglen, Co Armagh, an award-winning writer and a seasoned broadcaster. He is married to Brid, and has three children, Jack, Katie, and Grace.

He was a columnist for the British Medical Journal for 20 years and currently writes for GP, the leading newspaper for general practitioners in the UK. He has also been a columnist for the Lancet, the Journal of General Practice, the Belfast Telegraph and the Irish News. He wrote the entry on 'Sex' for The Oxford Companion to the Body. On Twitter he curates #Irishmed, a weekly tweetchat on all things medical, which has a global following. He also co-curates #WritersWise, a regular tweetchat for writers, with novelist Sharon Thompson.

He was the medical columnist for the BBC Radio Ulster Evening Extra 1996-98; presented the series Health-Check for Ulster TV in 2002, and was medical consultant for both series of Country Practice in 2000 and 2002 for BBC Northern Ireland. He is a member of the editorial board of the Hektoen International Medical Journal, Chicago.

His awards include Columnist of the Year at Irish Medical Media Awards 2003, Periodical Publishers Association of Great Britain 2006 and Medical Journalist's Society, London 2011, and Advancing Health through Media at the Zenith Global Healthcare Awards 2018.

He was shortlisted for the Michael McLaverty Short Story Competition in 2008.

Twitter: https://twitter.com/drlfarrell

To Brid, Jack, Katie, Gracie and Coco

I'd also like to dedicate this book to the late Lorna Markey. I worked with Lorna for 20 years, and she knew our patients and their seed, breed and generation better than any doctor. She was feisty and brave, yet unfailingly kind; *ar dheas Dé go raibh a anam.*

Acknowledgements

I'm indebted to many people; my English teachers at Abbey CBS Newry, Pat Mooney and the late Brother Magee, and my editors at the BMJ and GP, particularly Richard Smith, the late Ruth Holland, Linda Beauchamp, Fiona Godlee, Trevor Jackson, Richard Hurley, Bronagh Miskelly, Emma Bower and Neil Durham.

In particular, I'd like to thank Ruth Devlin and my daughter Grace for their help with the editing, and the Feldstein Literary Agency for their encouragement, enthusiasm, and good advice.

I'm also grateful to the people of Crossmaglen for their support throughout the years. When I started practice Dr Jack Crummie told me they were the best people in the world, and, as usual, he was absolutely right.

Published with permission of the British Medical Journal, GP magazine and the Journal of General Practice; almost seems like they were glad to see the back of me.

'I love Liam and his writing for three reasons. One, he tells it fearlessly like it is, as he is, and not under some sheepish pseudonym. Two, just because he tells it like it is, doesn't mean it's true. Like all great comic writers, he polishes a grain of truth until it's a pearl of pleasure and beautifully-crafted debauchery that still smells true. Three, unless he's been lying to me, Liam is a deeply flawed individual with a heart of gold whose life is even more interesting than the stuff he makes up.'

Dr Phil Hammond, author of 'Trust me, I'm a doctor' and Private Eye's 'MD' columnist

'Liam Farrell began to write a column for the BMJ after he won a competition when I was editing the journal, and his column proved so popular that he long outlasted me. Liam's is a unique voice that appealed very much to me and to his many BMJ readers. He combined insight, humour, and an often surreal style that inspired, provoked and entertained in equal measures.'

Richard Smith, BMJ editor-in-chief, 1991-2004

'Liam Farrell writes with razor sharp wit and allure. His personal account of his addiction is one of the most compelling I have ever read. In fact, it made me immediately phone the editor of the journal that published it to ask for Liam's contact details. I still get goose pimples thinking about that piece, years later.'

Dr Chris Smith, Managing Editor, The Naked Scientists www.thenakedscientists.com

Dr Liam Farrell has written for *GP* since 2002. In 2005 he was the first doctor to win columnist of the year in the Periodical Publishers Association (PPA) awards. He was also columnist of the year at the Medical Journalists' Association awards in 2011 where the judges praised his ability 'to convey so much information in a very funny short piece with a great punchline'. He has a loyal fanbase of *GP* readers who identify all too easily with his darkly humorous tales. A passionate defender of the NHS, he is unafraid to criticize government policy, from its 'naming and shaming' over GP cancer referrals to its covert NHS privatisation agenda.'

Neil Durham, editor, GP

Items should be returned on or before the last date shown below. Items not already requested by other borrowers may be renewed in person, in writing or by telephone. To renew, please quote the number on the barcode label. To renew online a PIN is required. This can be requested at your local library.
Renew online @ **www.dublincitypubliclibraries.ie**
Fines charged for overdue items will include postage incurred in recovery. Damage to or loss of items will be charged to the borrower.

Leabharlanna Poiblí Chathair Bhaile Átha Cliath
Dublin City Public Libraries

Dublin City
Baile Átha Cliath

Date Due	Date Due	Date Due

First published in 2018 by Dalzell Press.

Dalzell Press
54 Abbey Street
Bangor, N. Ireland
BT20 4JB

© Liam Farrell 2018

ISBN 978-0-9563864-6-5

All of the entries herein were previously published in the British Medical Journal, GP, or the Journal of Medical Practice, and are reprinted here with their permission.

Some names and identifying details have been changed to protect the privacy of individuals.

Table of Contents

'Are you the fucking doctor?' he asked.

I explained carefully, not wanting any mis-understanding, that I was just the ordinary doctor.

Introduction

The Ryanair attendant, desperation in his eyes, was trying to flog me a scratch card, while the gaudy blue and yellow paint was offending my sensibilities and making me nauseous. Only Ryanair could take this miracle and turn it to dross; this miracle of hurling a hundred tons of metal into the air and yet landing it safely again.

Ryanair may do it better than anyone else, but really, we are all guilty: we take the miracles of science for granted and then complain when science doesn't have all the answers. Of course, it is totally our fault for expecting that it should.

For most of the patients I see every day in the surgery, cold science and cool reason have only a minor part to play – there is a good reason why Mr Spock was not medical officer on the Enterprise. The emotional and vulnerable McCoy was a better choice – plus he had a little pen-thingy which was a cracking diagnostic aid.

Science needs a problem to solve; often we doctors do not actually know what the problem is, or who actually has the problem. No clinical textbook is of any use for these indecipherables and imponderables.

We doctors live on the cusp of uncertainties; we dance on the edge of knives. Science takes us only so far, but then the maps stop, ceding to the grey areas of intuition and imagination and feelings. Fortunately, these are powerful weapons; I learnt more about the human mind from Dostoyevsky's *Crime and Punishment* than I did from any psychiatry textbook.

Every one of us has suffered, so we can empathise with Van Gogh's self-portrait - the artist and the observer and the shared experience, the doctor and the patient and the mutual understanding. In contrast to the cold and hard-earned truths of scientific medicine, this is all vague and uncertain: it has to be learned by bitter experience; it can't be taught; it needs sensitivity and empathy.

I'm going out now to look at the sunset; it always makes me want to cry, especially when I am flying home with Ryanair.

Chapter 1

Transient pleasure, prolonged pain

I hope this book will make you smile, but in this first chapter there is no laughter, only pain and guilt. Perhaps it lends perspective to everything that follows; satire can be a cry for help, a shout of repressed pain, driven by fears and uncertainties, and the comic muse deflects tragedy just as the tragic muse embraces it.

I don't know how it started. I should have been happy; I had a steady and fulfilling job, I had a wife and three children whom I loved and who loved me, I had many good friends. I lived in a beautiful home.

I was working very hard, and the work kept piling up. I was on duty every second night for the practice, was writing columns for four magazines and newspapers, all with different readerships, and had started my own medical newspaper. I was also a postgraduate tutor in care of the dying and had been lecturing and writing for years how doctors should not be afraid of using morphine; that fear of its side-effects was depriving patients of necessary pain-relief.

But none of these are excuses, only background.

For such a catastrophic turning point in my life, I have no memory of the first time I injected myself with morphine. Somewhere, somehow, I obviously thought I would try it myself, see what it was like; I learned that lesson the hard way. I didn't become a stranger to myself, but rather a different me, perhaps a truer, more basic me, veneers of conscience and morals and consideration for others ripped away, all for that single brief glorious rush. It was a harsh time, but, I always remember, harsher for Brid and for those who cared about me.

11

Despite making a career as a writer, I have had no desire to write about my addiction, so this piece has been my only effort. I sat down one night and wrote it in one sitting, as a warning to others, and a reminder to myself what a horrible, squalid, selfish little vice it is.

The vein stands up proudly. It's good to look at, it's inviting. The tourniquet is satisfyingly tight, the syringe waits like a shark on the bedside table, the new orange needle catches a glint of light, a silver gleam of expectancy, hungry for the vein; one of the small benefits of being a doctor and an addict is that new and clean needles are easily available, and the risk of AIDS and hepatitis B or C and other infections is accordingly low. New needles also won't have been blunted by repeated use. I had used a bigger green needle to draw up the drug, a needle that can reach right to the bottom of the ampoule, so that not one drop will be missed. I use an orange needle for the actual injection because it is of smaller bore and will penetrate the skin much more easily, with less trauma, and will leave less visible evidence.

Beside the syringe lies the pack of Cyclimorph, a combination of morphine and cyclizine, empty now, and ominous, a small harbinger of doom. The particular colour of the red and blue packaging is like a beacon to me; when I see those colours alarm bells go off in my head, if a pack was lying by the side of the road a mile away I would spot it immediately. At this moment I don't care that it's my last dose; the future, and the price I am going to have to inevitably pay, is irrelevant. I'm living in the now, isn't that the secret of happiness, and everything is focused on my preparations.

The discarded packaging of the needles, ampoules and syringe lie in a tidy little pile. I put the guard back on the green needle and set it beside the empty ampoule; these need more careful attention, as discarded needles can turn up anywhere and ampoules can shatter easily and leave small but sharp shards of glass. The detritus has to be kept together, so that it can be secretly disposed of; secrecy is paramount, nobody can know, nobody can suspect. If I wait till after I've used, I may forget, or become too casual, and leave some evidence behind. I don't want questions I don't want challenges, I don't want tough love, I don't want people who care about me, I want the drug.

Everything is quiet, the doors are closed, the curtains pulled, all is dark except for the bedside lamp, just bright enough to see what I'm doing, a small island of light in this world I have created for myself, a world of shadows and self-destruction. I am alone in the house, just the way I have planned it; there is no glamour here, no drama, no heroin chic, no grand passion, no tortured artistic sensibility, it's just a selfish, venal, deceitful, squalid, solitary vice.

I roll the vein lightly with my forefinger, testing the bounce, no, much more than that, not just testing it, enjoying the bounce; the vein you can feel is more reliable than the vein you can see. The vein is sweetly engorged, sensual, and will be easy to access, little chance of missing the vein and the drug leaking into the subcutaneous tissues, which would leave a painful and visible bruise and, even worse, would mean losing some of the drug. The vein I have selected is on my right forearm, on the inner surface. As I am right-handed, my left arm is a better choice, but after months of injecting, the larger veins there have collapsed, and the only veins that remain visible are thin and thready and would be unreliable. I still have some attractively superficial veins on the back of my left hand which would be easy to access, but the marks there will be too easy to see. The hand veins can wait for the time when I become more desperate; their day of service will come, and come soon.

My right forearm is doubly awkward, as not only will I have to use my clumsier left hand to access the vein, but also the skin on the inner surface of the arm is paler and will show up marks much more vividly, especially if something goes wrong and I bruise excessively. I am pale-skinned at the best of times, and months of regular using has turned me wraith-like; I've seen recent photos, I look detached, like a ghost.

But this vein looks good, not only is it visible and easily palpable, but it is also near a junction, which usually means that it is tethered down by subcutaneous tissues and shouldn't move around too much; veins can be capricious, as if they have a mind of their own and sometimes seem to deliberately wriggle away from the needle. I have also become more skilled even with my left hand, so it shouldn't be hard to hit; I am confident.

Of course, even if I do bruise, I can always wear long sleeves; why should anyone be suspicious enough to want to inspect my arms? It isn't any of their business, it's my problem, I'll handle it myself. Who do they think they are, interfering, are they perfect? Nobody asked them.

I lift the syringe, holding it up to the light, admiring the liquid clarity of the drug. I flick the syringe to get rid of any air-bubbles; this is just another small piece of the ritual, small air-bubbles aren't dangerous. I check the needle; it is bevelled, and I want the bevel on the down-side of the needle, so it will be less likely to pass through the vein and out the other side. I line up the needle along the length of the vein and push it in. The needle penetrates the skin easily and painlessly; like a kiss, just a moment's resistance in the subcutaneous tissues till I feel it push through the wall of the vein. Yes, that's it, perfect; I draw back on the syringe to confirm I am in the vein. The dark blood froths satisfyingly back into the syringe, a plume of red billowing into the clear liquid of the drug, intoxicating to look at, an unforgettable image, I have hit the mother-lode, a red flag signalling go; is it joy I feel, or is it more like relief? Joy is too decent an emotion for something like this.

Sometimes, even when I am sure I am in the vein, only a trickle of blood comes back. This might mean that the needle is outside the vein, probably gone through it; but it might also mean that the vein has a small lumen and I could still go ahead. I am then faced with an urgent decision. Do I try to deliver the drug? If I do, and I'm not in the vein, I'll feel the resistance, the drug won't go in easily, and I'll see a little dimple appear at the injection site, a hateful little thing which signifies trouble and complications and delay in getting the drug. Then I'll have no choice, I'll have to pull out the needle. Morphine in the tissues is painful and will leave a big bruise. Even worse, I'll have lost some of the drug; that hateful little dimple represents a lost rush. Common-sense would dictate I stop at once and start again; step back from the ritual, be patient, take out the needle, put pressure on the site to limit the bleeding and bruising, be sensible, start all over again, find another vein. But it's hard when I'm so close, and addicts aren't patient, I want the drug now.

And if I do have to try again, there is a danger that the blood which has trickled back will clot in the syringe, I may lose the drug, suddenly I am in a panic; quick, decide if I need to decant the drug into the spare syringe I have brought, as the clot would most likely occur in the syringe's nozzle, but then I'll probably lose some of the drug in the transfer, not much, but I don't want to lose

15

any of the drug, quick, strap on the tourniquet again, quick, quick, find another vein, anywhere, who cares if it's a hand vein, who cares if it bruises and everyone can see it, quick, quick, it's not the leisurely and pleasurable stalk I'd enjoyed just a few minutes before. When I pull out the needle, it may ooze blood, stain and spot the bed-clothes, stain my shirt, I usually wear dark clothes just in case, but pressure with a tissue is a secondary issue now, I mustn't lose the drug. I throw away the needle, I'll just have to remember to look for it later. I have to find a vein and access it before I lose the drug, whatever I do I mustn't lose the drug, I mustn't lose the drug. And in that panic I may have trouble finding a vein, I may have to try a number of times, each time in increasing desperation, needles and blood and blood-stained tissues everywhere, sometimes I end up sticking in needles almost at random where I think a vein should be, there's bound to be a vein in there somewhere, isn't there, and each attempt leaving a bloody bruise.

But this time I am certain; the blood has bubbled freely and easily back into the syringe and there is no doubt I am in the vein.

Everything is ready, all my careful planning has brought me successfully to this point. The pleasure of the anticipation is almost spent. Call me Pavlov's addict; getting my hands on the new pack of Cyclimorph, arranging things carefully that I am alone and won't be disturbed, assembling all the required paraphernalia, the tourniquet, a reliable one that won't snap open when I tighten it but be easy to release when the needle is in the vein, two two-ml syringes, the extra one in case I miss the vein and the first syringe looks in danger of clotting, two green needles and five or six orange needles, dark tissue paper, preferably, or if not a dark towel, then closing the door, looping the tourniquet round my arm and pulling it tight, seeing a suitable vein rise up, touching it, feeling it, taking the ampoule out of the pack, cracking open the ampoule, fitting the needle on the syringe, feeling the scrape of the green needle on the bottom of the ampoule, drawing up the drug, all these things become a pleasure.

I've tried other injecting other drugs which I knew wouldn't provide any rush; hydrocortisone, diazepam, partly out of curiosity but also to satisfy these learned pleasures. The diazepam made me drowsy and the hydrocortisone gave me a prickling sensation in the perineum; I only tried it once.

Even when I'm not about to use I will catch myself looking at a vein in my hands and arms, rubbing my fingers over it speculatively. I'll notice other peoples' veins too; even having a drink with friends, I'd be observing who has prominent veins. This might partly, a very small part, I admit, be a hangover from my days as medical student and learning how to set up intravenous fluids; a patient with big, prominent cord-like veins could be sorted in moments, a patient with tubby arms and veins buried in layers of subcutaneous fat could be a problem.

I slip off the tourniquet and slowly press the plunger fully in; the drug goes in easily, no sense of resistance that might suggest the vein wasn't patent.

I need to act quickly now to prepare for the rush, to experience it fully; I don't want any outside stimuli which might interfere with the consummation. My movements are practiced; I whip out the needle, and throw the syringe away, I'll pick it up later, I've no time to set it aside carefully. I press my left hand firmly on the site with a dark red paper tissue. A white tissue would show up the blood too obviously and might turn up somewhere inconvenient and hard to explain away. The firm pressure will restrict localized bruising and make the injection site less easy to spot, if someone was looking for it. There will inevitably be a mark of some sort, but I hope nothing too obvious, and as everything has gone smoothly it should clear up in a few days. Firm pressure will also help keep the vein patent for future use, so I'll keep the pressure on even during the rush.

I take off my glasses, switch off the light, lie back and close my eyes. Alone in the dark, in my own little bubble, no light, no noise, I wait.

Within seconds, I feel the rush coming on, firstly a tingle coming up my right arm, then a wonderful warm tidal wave stroking my whole skin, my whole body; it seems to find a centre deep within my chest. I try to savour each moment, each instant, but just as quickly as it comes it is gone; that's it, done, all over, it lasted a few breaths at most.

I'm disappointed it's over and wish I could turn back time a few seconds. I also feel dissatisfied, a bit cheated; the rush wasn't quite as good as I hoped it would be, because it is only a few hours since I last used. I wish I'd held off for a few hours, then I'd still have the drug, and the rush would have been better.

I am slightly sedated but not overly so. I could walk down the street and exchange greetings and take part in a normal conversation, and even those who knew me well might not be able to detect that something was different, something was very wrong; my voice might be deeper, my pupils dilated, but nothing very obvious. My wife would know, but she might not challenge me; I'll meet any challenge with hostility.

I am comfortable and relaxed; the drug makes me feel pleasantly languid, like I'm wrapped in cotton wool. Morphine dries me up. My mouth is dry, my nose won't run, my bowels won't move, it's hard to pass urine and I won't get any erections. I feel the morphine itch, but it's not distressing, just asking for an agreeable scratch.

But even at this stage, even so soon after injecting, not much more than a few minutes, reality starts to pull me back in. The fog lifts, the modest euphoria which lingers after the rush begins to leak away. I start to worry about getting rid of the evidence. I get up, and first of all look on the floor for the syringe I hastily discarded. For this I need to turn on the wall lights, the glare harsh and unforgiving on the little piles of detritus. I stand blinking in the light, but the syringe is easy to find on this occasion, sticking point down in the carpet, as if it was a little dart. Sometimes I am not so lucky; the syringes can hide themselves under beds, behind books, and demand minutes of anxious searching and scrabbling. Sometimes I don't find them, and they lie in wait like predators, choosing their moment to turn up.

I collect all the paraphernalia, the packaging and the sharps, to put them somewhere safe so I can dispose of them later; the paper stuff can go in the normal rubbish, hidden in a plastic bag, secreted at the bottom of the bin. In a few days I'll take the needles and empty ampoules into the surgery, where there is a special sharps box for safe disposal. I check the floor again carefully to make sure nothing has dropped. Often, I miss something and leave evidence, the syringe wrapping, a blood-stained tissue, the top of an ampoule, the occasional needle. If I've had trouble finding a vein, I may have had to use four or five needles and together with the panic this brings on, it's easy to lose count and miss one.

I am becoming more aware that that was my last ampoule of Cyclimorph. I already knew this, of course, but I had put off the evil day of facing up to it.

I have no more supplies of the drug, so withdrawal effects are inevitable. I've been through morphine withdrawal symptoms before and it was pitiless; I had read about it, of course, and I knew it was unpleasant, but nothing could have prepared me for how cruel it was, and having to go through it again frightens me. I know theoretically that withdrawal effects should not begin until about six to eight hours after the last dose, but such is my fear of withdrawal that I begin to feel uncomfortable after only a few hours.

Long before the symptoms start I can't settle, I know what is to come, it hangs over me like a weight. The world seems to be painted grey, I start to feel cold and sweaty. I feel a draught from the window; just a draught, it would make even a normal person shiver, but it has more significance to me. Is it more than a draught, is it making me shiver because the withdrawal effects are starting? I know in theory there should be a few hours yet before their onset, but knowing this is no defence. My skin feels prickly and uncomfortable, the hairs are standing up, which is why they call it going cold turkey; or maybe I just think I am starting to feel that way, maybe it is my fear playing tricks. I have no defence. I am frightened and alone, facing into the oncoming storm, and it is all my own fault, all my own work. My fear is rising up to choke me.

I have looked it up, I have the medications which in theory should help alleviate the symptoms; loperamide for the diarrhoea, diazepam for the anxiety, mefenamic acid for the muscle cramps. But I also know from previous experience that they will have only a minimal effect.

As each hour passes the symptoms get worse; they are real now, and accompanied by muscle pains and abdominal cramps and diarrhoea and fatigue. I am cold, then hot, my skin rasps and prickles and burns. My nose is dripping constantly, my eyes water, I dab at them repeatedly with a paper tissue and by the end my eyes and nose will be red and raw. I glimpse myself in a mirror, my face is white, except for my cheeks, which are flushed bright red, beads of sweat on my forehead. I know that, unlike alcohol and benzodiazepine withdrawal, there is no significant medical risk and individually the physical symptoms aren't that bad, no worse than a bad flu. Put me in a warm room, with plenty of fluids, and they'd be tolerable.

But the anxiety, the anxiety and the fear, is overwhelming; I am like a vibrating string. I cannot sit for even a moment without having to get up. Once up I have to sit down again. I try to go to bed, but I can't get comfortable, I thrash and turn every second of every minute of every hour. The sheets are rough and unpleasant against my skin and my sweat soon turns them damp and rank. And I know this will continue for the next forty-eight hours at least. Only forty-eight hours, only two days, I tell myself, doesn't sound very long, someone take this cup away from me. I've been ill before, I've had injuries before, I've had bad times before, and I've been able to handle them, able to put my head down and struggle on, but nothing has ever unmanned me like withdrawal, nothing has ever left me so scared, so lacking in courage, nothing has ever beaten down my resistance like this, there is no way out, no way to escape.

Except to take another dose, which would relieve all the symptoms instantly, it would be like a miracle. But I don't have another dose and it's too late to get any more. And if I did, I'd only be postponing the ordeal. I've had the pleasure, and now I have to pay the price. The preparation was elaborate and the consequences prolonged and grim, yet the gratification was only fleeting; it is a transaction that makes no sense, a fool's bargain, a kind of madness. I am dancing between blades, one of them soft and desirable, and the other harsh and bitter; they both cut deep and take chunks of my spirit away each time. This is over-dramatizing it, there is no point to this, I am just a miserable damp heap of guilt and self-pity and self-loathing.

How did it come to this, I ask myself again and again, how did I let this happen to me? My mind races; I went through withdrawal before, vowed it would never happen again, that this time I would stay clean. Why did I have to start using again and get myself into this mess? And when I did start again why did not I show some self-control and use on an occasional basis, once a week or once a month, where I wouldn't have developed a physical addiction again? And why did I have to use that last packet so quickly? There are five ampoules in each pack of Cyclimorph, I should have been able to string it out over at least three days. Even five days; one dose every night would have been feasible, the withdrawal effects might have been coming on, but they would be quite tolerable if I knew I had a supply and that within a short time not only would they be banished completely but that I'd be getting the drug.

But that's not how my addiction works. After I've used, even just a few hours, somewhere deep in my mind, the merest hint of a thought will come to me about using again. The pack of Cyclimorph, that wonderful red-and-blue pack, is sitting somewhere, hidden away securely, but it's calling to me, a whispering siren, eating away at my resistance. Even by the perverted laws of an addict's world, this makes no sense; I know that the rush won't be as good because I've used so recently, I know the longer I hold off, the greater the rush will be, but knowing my enemy is no advantage to me, and soon the ritual has started again, soon I'm closing the doors, taking out the ampoule and cracking it open and drawing up the drug. Once I even think, even the briefest passing thought, once I think of using again I can't get it out of my head, and the deal is as good as done, and a pack of five that should have lasted me three days or more is gone in less than twenty-four hours.

Scared and alone, I shiver and sweat, and try to count down the minutes. I drink as much fluids as I can, staying well hydrated can help the symptoms, though I feel nauseated. Some junkies vomit copiously during cold turkey but that's not how it affects me; neither do I hallucinate, and I don't have nightmares. I have no appetite, when I do force myself to eat I have no sense of taste. Since I became an addict I've lost weight; taking the drug removes my appetite, going through withdrawal removes my appetite. I love reading, but I'm too distracted to concentrate, and my eyes are watering so much my vision is blurred, I look like I've been crying, and my emotions are so labile I do burst into tears regularly, great gusts of tears, of self-pity. Don't feel sorry for me, I don't deserve it, I am only crying for myself.

I switch on the television; George of the Jungle is playing, a comedy, but I am far away from laughter. I try to stay with the movie for a few minutes, but I find sitting tiring; I can't hold my head up, and I slump forward, I have to get up and walk around. This is going to destroy me.

I go for a walk outside, trying to distract myself, take my mind of it, exercise is supposed to help the symptoms, use up some of that adrenaline that is surging round my body, protesting and looking for a release; it has been suppressed for a long time by the activation of the morphine receptors, now the dam has cracked and it is pouring out vindictively, seeking justice, seeking revenge. After crime comes the punishment. I am desperately tired, dragging one leg after the other. But even though it's a fine warm day, the sun shining in an all-blue sky, everyone else in t-shirts and summer clothes, it's much too cold for me. The faintest breeze is uncomfortable; I have a big coat on, but I am sweating underneath it, a cold, cold sweat. I can't stay out for long anyway in case I get another episode of diarrhoea.

I am an outcast; I see a father walking along the roadside, holding his children by the hand. It's like a knife, a small parcel of anguish, why can't I be like that, be a normal dad, with normal interests and normal concerns. I remember it, I remember walks and family picnics, birthdays, holidays, Christmas. The memories seem to come from a far distance, a long-lost place. I've sent this happiness, this contentment, away from me. The normal world is a rainbow of colours, mine is dull and grey. Why can't I be like that still, how did I lose it? It's a selfish ordeal, I'm drowning, too immersed in my own misery to think about the people I am hurting, my wife, my children. 'A devil in the house,' my wife calls it, no matter how many times she tries to push it out it keeps on getting back in again. The drug has come between us, has ruptured that bond, that presumption that we were a couple and a family, that we would meet everything together and handle it together. I have betrayed the trust, I have promised her again and again that I would stop, that no, I'm not acting strangely and no, I haven't used and no, there's nothing wrong with my voice, and yes, I'm clean, that this was definitely the last time, but I'm like all addicts; you know I'm lying because my lips are moving.

And I get angry when my lies are challenged, when she asks about a blood-stained tissue, or wants to see my arms to check for bruises, or finds a stray needle or empty ampoule. I make up some story, try to explain it away, I had a blood test today, or I banged my arm on the car door, the ampoule must have been there from a few months ago, it sounds stupid even as I'm saying it, but it's all I've got. What about the kids, she asks, supposing Jack or Katie or Gracie had hurt themselves on that needle, how would you feel, do you not consider them? I have no answer, I think I care, but the drug comes first every time.

I check the time constantly, willing the minutes to pass. Forty-eight hours, I tell myself, only forty-eight hours to get through, then things will get easier and I'll know the worst is over, but only a few hours have gone, the time drags, the seconds inch along. I lie down again. I get up again, double up with a spasm of abdominal pain, go to the kitchen to drink some water, endure yet another episode of diarrhoea. I am dirty and sweaty, I take a bath, which helps warm me up, but I am too agitated to stay in it for long and getting out of a warm water is a shock; I am instantly freezing, I scrub myself urgently dry.

And then the first night; I dread the night, darkness was my friend, but now the hours stretch ahead of me, there will be no relief, no oasis, just a long darkness.

But, I promise to myself, this is the last time. This is definitely the last time, I won't put myself through this ordeal again; this time I'll stay clean. I promise.

As I write this, I'm over ten years clean, and grateful to the many good people who helped me; when you are fighting for your life you need your family and friends to believe in you. And to the still-suffering addict out there, I say this; there is a rich life waiting for you, you can get better.

Chapter 2

Love and Sex

I still remember the first time I put on a white coat and hung a stethoscope around my neck; a bit like the first time I had sex, although not as sweaty and with less protection, and with more ridicule from those more experienced; je ne regrette rien, I say, good sex may be great, but bad sex is still good.

The Christmas issue of the BMJ is always off-beat, and that year they commissioned seven highly-regarded doctors to write an academic review of the positive aspects of the Seven Deadly Sins I was allocated Lust, for some unknown reason.

Soon after I was commissioned to write the entry on Sex for the Oxford Companion to the Body. I had become typecast as an expert on sex, and it's been hard to shake off this reputation.

Casablanca

BMJ 11 August 2010

Of all the gin joints, in all the towns, in all the world . . . but if you watch the skies for long enough, I reflected, sooner or later an attractive new planet will swim into your ken. Bogart would have known the feeling; tall and willowy, she was the kind of woman who made you suspect that testosterone deficiency was yet another illusory drug company construct rather than a real disease.

'You requested a second opinion on Mrs Murphy,' she said, lips pouting.

'Let's drive,' I said.

Leaving town, I saw three thugs harassing an old lady in a wheelchair. I chased them away, giving one a good clip on the ear.

'*Pour encourager les autres,*' I explained, in my best Serge Gainsbourg.

'*Vous parlez Français?*' she said, Jane Birkin metaphorically riding up on a scooter.

'*Un petit peu,*' I said modestly.

We were driving along a sun-dappled country road past genetically modified cows, when I braked suddenly; before she could protest I was already returning to the car, cradling a tiny kitten in my arms.

'The poor wee thing was abandoned in the middle of the road,' I said, wrapping the kitten in a blanket improvised from an obsolete swine flu protective suit (we have only thousands left), 'but I know a little gal who lost a puppy a few weeks ago; she'll give her a good home.'

At the house (luckily Mrs Murphy's buxom niece Sally was not around; that could have been awkward—I hate women fighting over me), she confirmed my diagnosis. 'Your doctor was right,' she said, 'nothing functional or airy fairy here, definitely a case of systemic lupus erythematosus!'

'Isn't he always,' said Mrs Murphy, handing over her protection money. I palmed the cash and slipped her some antibiotics.

On the way back I stopped, taking out my mandolin and a hamper full of smoked salmon and champagne. 'Had we but all the earth and time / Then Lady, coyness were no crime,' I whispered. Her lips tasted of oranges and wine, and we made love on a bed of autumn leaves and magic mushrooms, her soft cries of ecstasy counterpointed by the hungry mewing of the kitten.

'My Achilles,' she murmured throatily, 'Will I see you tonight?'

'I never plan that far ahead,' I said.

'What kind of doctor are you?' she wondered.

'A doctor like any other,' I said, 'Only more so.'

Love, a weakness?

GP 17 October 2012

I like to consider myself widely read, but I have to admit that Fifty Shades of Grey has not yet graced my bookshelf.

I understand that its themes are the joys of love, sadomasochism and sexual perversity, but I'm too old for that stuff. Been there, done that, wore the very sweaty T-shirt, preferred doing it to reading about it, and I remember well the first time I had sex; I still have the receipt.

Call me cynical, but love is a weakness, something to exploit in others, not to sink into like quicksand. As Groucho said in *A Day at the Races*: 'Have the florist send some roses to Mrs Upjohn, and write 'Emily, I love you' on the back of the bill.'

Love can be inconvenient and manipulative as well.

'I love you, doctor,' she said, her eyes shining (though maybe that was due to the drugs). I hasten to add that this incident happened long, long ago, when I was young and gorgeous. I must also admit I prefer young women, the younger the better, but that is purely because their medical histories are shorter.

'And do you love me?' she asked.

'As a secular humanist,' I extemporised, not wanting to be unnecessarily brusque and hurtful. 'We believe in loving everyone for their own sake and not as per the instruction of some imaginary mythical being. But it's a global thing, you understand, and shouldn't be taken personally.'

'But the way you touched me just now, I definitely felt something,' she said.

'Taking your BP cannot in any way be construed as an erotic activity,' I replied, getting ready to push the emergency button and remembering that we hadn't actually got around to connecting it up. 'Any physical contact was a medical necessity.'

'You can't hide your feelings,' she said.

'Madame,' I said. 'My feelings are irrelevant. From your perspective, I am not a man, I am a doctor. You may consider me an asexual robot, the damnably handsome kind.'

'So our love can never be,' she said.

'Never,' I agreed.

'Oh well,' she said. 'Can I have some antibiotics then?'

'Sure,' I said, feeling relieved and yet manipulated.

Sex and prostate cancer; what they don't want you to know

GP 10 November 2011

'I'm worried,' said Joe. Joe is always worried, but sometimes his worries can be entertaining, so I put on my interested expression.

'I read in the Daily Mail' he said, 'That more than three eggs each week greatly increases the risk of prostate cancer.'

'Ah yes, indeed, the Daily Mail,' I said, saying it like I'd just trod in something, 'I've written columns for what we medical folk like to call the lay press, and I understand their priorities. The average newspaper is uninterested in cold hard facts about health, and prefers instead attention-grabbing headlines. This problem is compounded by researchers desperately looking for headlines themselves, so that they get their grants and drinking money beefed up.'

'But what about the eggs?' said Joe.

'Eggs always seem to get a bad rap,' I said. 'When I was a medical student eggs were public enemy number one due to their cholesterol content. Until recently, the British Heart Foundation recommended eating no more than three a week because of fears that they raised the risk of heart attacks and strokes. It only dropped the recommendation in 2007 after evidence emerged that very little of the cholesterol contained in eggs enters the bloodstream. These fashions come and go; eat away, and enjoy.'

'I'm still worried,' he said.

'That's what doctors are for,' I said gaily, 'And I have the perfect remedy for your concerns; patient education is always of prime importance to The Good Doctor. A report from the British Journal of Urology suggested that men who ejaculated more than five times each week in their 20s, 30s, and 40s reduced their risk of developing prostate cancer by a third. Of course, further research is needed, you know how guys love to boast, and anyway these were Australians.'

'Five times each week,' he mused. 'But I'm not married.'

'Let's be frank here, we're both men of the world,' I said. 'There's nothing wrong with masturbation, though I understand it's not exactly the Capulets and the Montagues, is it? And by the way, we prefer the term, 'Solitary recreation."

'Solitary recreation,' he said slowly, 'But that will make it safe to eat eggs?'

'Every time you eat an egg …,' I said encouragingly.

'If it's for the good of my health,' he said, visibly steeling himself. 'That's a sacrifice I'm willing to make.'

Joe returned a month later, oily with self-satisfaction. An oily Joe is a dangerous Joe; it's like when Frankenstein was happy, playing with the little girl, not the best time to go near him with a torch.

'That advice you gave me,' he purred. 'It was great stuff altogether.'

'And what advice was this?' I asked, with some trepidation.

'Don't you remember,' he said. 'You encouraged me to start masturbating, or should I say, indulging in 'solitary recreation."

'I don't recall being quite so directive,' I said carefully, 'I merely referred to a report from the British Journal of Urology. I didn't recommend you start making out like the Duracell Bunny.'

'Amounts to the same thing,' he said. 'Anyway, I've been talking about it with my mates and they've all started it too.'

He has actually admitted masturbating to his mates, I thought; some relationships are a bit too close for comfort.

'And then we thought, hey, we shouldn't be selfish and keep this important breakthrough to ourselves, this concerns everyone, it's a public health issue; all that advertising about prostate cancer awareness, yet the positive health benefits of masturbation, excuse me, solitary recreation, are never emphasised.'

'Health promotion does, by tradition, have a rather puritanical outlook,' I admitted.

'This is our chance to change attitudes,' he said passionately. 'To drag masturbation, I mean, solitary recreation, out of the closet. We're not gonna be ashamed anymore, so we're starting a Facebook page and a Twitter campaign and we're going worldwide, with flag days, celebrity endorsements, sponsored walks to Machu Picchu, the whole hog. And a naked calendar; purely for fundraising purposes, of course, it's not that we actually like getting our kit off in public, is it?'

'And you'll have a willing audience,' I said, by now fascinated at where this was going. 'To paraphrase George Bernard Shaw, 98 per cent of men are practising prostatic cancer prevention and the other 2 per cent are liars.'

'That's the spirit,' he said. 'I really feel I can make a difference, I'm energised, I'm ... '

'All pumped up?' I suggested.

'Exactly,' he said. 'There was something missing in my life, but now I have a goal, I have something worth fighting for. And if I fail, does that make my deeds any less valorous?'

The words rose unbidden, the Blues Brothers sitting on my shoulder.

'You're on an emission from God,' I said.

When bad news is actually good news

GP 30 October 2015

I rode that surgery like it was a great black stallion. Every patient was much more than just a life-story, more an epic poem, full of tragedy and triumph, good and evil, despair and hope, and all misfortunes and predicaments were trampled to dust under the iron-shod hooves of my mighty steed.

Then Joe came in, yet again, and at once I was dwindled. My struggle no longer heroic, but instead a Slough of Despond of whiny kids and grumpy old men and sick certs and passport forms and antibiotics and sleeping tablets, and me a deluded old knight astride a moth-eaten Rozinante.

Joe has that effect on me, my golden morning turned to dross, like clouds covering the sun, or switching on Sky Sports and finding the live match is West Brom vs Stoke City; we usually get along best when neither of us is actually listening fully to what the other is saying.

But even on a moonless night there are stars; Joe had dysuria, unusual in young men, and more diverting than his usual complaints, like the exhaustive and rather creepy diary he keeps on the tone, shape, consistency, and colour of his bowel movements.

Careful yet sensitive questioning (because I am sometimes A Good Doctor) revealed (via the usual euphemisms) that Joe had had unprotected sex, and not (this was the real killer) in the usual solitary manner, but with an actual real person, a lady.

Despite my astonishment and revulsion and fascination, however, I didn't renege on my clinical responsibilities.

'Joe, you idiot,' I said, breaking it to him gently. 'You have a sexually transmitted disease.'

Most people would not consider this to be good news, but so dreary has Joe's mother-dominated lifestyle been, with such an unyielding absence of novelty, that this shadow also meant a light.

'Have I really?' he said (was that tear in his eye?). 'Gosh, I can't wait to tweet about it.'

To Joe, it was validation, proof, like getting a certificate which said, 'You have engaged in sexual activity and are therefore not irredeemably repulsive'.

When an STD is the highlight of your life…

Play up, play up and play the game

GP 2 November 2012

General practice is a broad church, with room for all body shapes, varieties and temperaments.

This is usually a good thing for our patients, as it gives them a choice. If they want a leisurely, throw-another-log-on-the-fire chat, they may prefer to see my partner. If they want it quick, I'm their man. It's not that I want to rush them out, you understand, it's just that I'm so eager to see the next patient.

The same goes for sexuality; my father's house has many mansions. I'm vaguely heterosexual myself, but not absolutely certain. When I was young and beautiful and enjoyed experimentation, some Cossacks whistled at me once, and I have hazy memories of someone with long hair at Woodstock; I had the kind of body that appealed to both persuasions.

But our hierarchy may not be so flexible. A senior member of the Royal College of General Practitioners was recently criticised for advising membership candidates to act 'less gay', when presenting for examination: deepen your voice, stand straighter, comb your hair, walk like John Wayne and talk like a redneck.

I think the criticisms were unfair; this was simply giving candidates a helpful steer. The upper echelons of medicine have never been known for their liberal tendencies, and when we are young and vulnerable we have to follow the rules and play the game. If that means acting like a square for a few hours, it's a small sacrifice to make. Once inside the golden door we can let it all hang out, baby.

But our increasingly heterogeneous profession can also make things a bit confusing. Recently a young colleague introduced me to his partner, which I found rather ambiguous.

'Practice or bedroom?' I had to ask. I like clarity, because one is then less likely to cause unintentional offence; intentional offence is much more satisfying.

'Both,' he said, as the two of them shared an intimate smirk. 'We like to practise a couple of times each day.' That's cool with me. I always like to think I am down with the kids, and I believe sexuality should remain a private affair.

Behind closed doors, it's just me and thousands of people on the internet.

Ulysses

BMJ 11 February 2009

I have been feeling more and more isolated, though I'm sure that the motives of Pele and Stirling Moss were admirable. All those soft-focused ads about what are coyly termed intimacy issues I could only gaze at covetously, knowing that I'd never belong to that blissful utopia of well preserved, handsome couples wandering dreamy eyed into the sunset—an Elysium where sex is never down and back-seat dirty.

The bandwagon of effete Western decadence had started to roll, the emperor's drunken soldiery were abed, and increasingly I was forced underground, yearning for that kinder, gentler time, that time of pre-Raphaelite innocence when I was a happy, horny guy, blithely exercising the *droit de seignur* befitting a scion of our ancient and aristocratic profession.

But I still couldn't escape it. 'Men's Health' was in my face everywhere, and like any self-respecting disease awareness campaign it was bankrolled and driven headlong by the drug industry. Check out any magazine or symposium on men's health and sooner or later there'll be an article on erectile dysfunction and a little footnote that the magazine or symposium is sponsored by one of the relevant drug companies, men's health being the Trojan horse from which they will flog their undoubtedly effective (so I'm told) wares.

Women's health is multifaceted and nuanced: breast disease, osteoporosis, menopausal disorders, the importance of lifestyle, and quality of life issues, including art and literature and the pursuit of happiness and understanding the beauty and fragility of the universe.

Men's health, by brutal contrast, is crude and insulting in its simplicity; is Ermintrude cranking or not? Men's health has become synonymous with erectile dysfunction. Anything else is just a smokescreen, nothing else matters to us, it's the only thing we care about—a demeaning stereotype that reduces our infinite humanity to the most primal Darwinian drives.

But as the great Richard Gordon said, you can't lead a gift horse to water and then look up its arse. The horse

36

has already penetrated the walls, and Ulysses, Diomedes, Viagra, Levitra, and Cialis are rampant in the city, violating the women, laying ruin the temples of Apollo, setting high Pergamon aflame, and hurling down the topmost towers of Ilium.

And relentlessly undermining the men's confidence.

L is for Lust

BMJ 21 December 1996

Lust does not appear in Index Medicus or Medline. We in the medical profession pretend that the most atavistic and implacable of all forces does not exist, though our colleagues in the clergy consider it the deadliest of all the deadly sins.

What, then, is lust? Like any good Irishman, shuddering with repressed Catholic guilt and Victorian prudery, I interpret lust as unfettered sexual desire, and not as some wishy-washy Van Goghian lust for life in general; as Jenny Diver screeched triumphantly in Brecht's *The Threepenny Opera*, 'Sexual obsession hath him in thrall.' In truth, our primal drives offer us little choice; we must see our descendants thrive and our genes become immortal.

But Mother Nature has been capriciously kind and has given us this irresistible imperative with a twinkle in her eye. Procreating is fun, great fun, though archaeologists now say that for the past few million years humans have consciously separated sex from reproduction; fortunately sex, even without procreation, is still great fun. Even bad sex is still good.

Lust drives us to create, to achieve, to make ourselves as attractive as possible; whether our dick substitute is a big shiny car or the tenderest love poem or the most outre art nouveau is simply a matter of taste—we are combing our peacock plumage with different strokes. But there is a snake in our garden of Eden, the serpent of sociocultural patterns which trammel this rich creative force into the bottlenecks of monogamy and sterility.

Imagine driving down the motorway in a Porsche and encountering a 30 mph zone; how do you restrain the six tons of throbbing horsepower between your legs? What congealing effect will it have on your spirit?

This is in regrettable contrast with the happy sexuality of other mammals, where sex is governed only by the availability of the female. The unfortunate female human who engages in sex without emotional involvement has been shown to feel vulnerable and this emotional vulnerability increases with the number of partners.[2] But could it be our society and its legacy of sexual limitation and equivocal morality which is the real cause of this vulnerability?

But even unsatisfied lust may have its good points. When Yeats, only 23, fell in unrequited love with Maud Gonne, his loss inspired the greatest body of love poetry in the English language; the anguish, the ruin, the grief, the lurching between melancholy and despair, 'It had become a glimmering girl/With apple-blossom in her hair/Who called me by my name and ran/And faded in the brightening air.'

Would a few good hard shags right at the start of their relationship have deprived us of these sublime and unforgettable verses? As Balzac said (afterwards), 'There goes another great novel.'

My role model

BMJ 20 June 1998

We are none of us saints, and a veneer of sophistication and restraint is all that lies between us and the unbridled satiation of our most venal appetites and our most primitive drives; to eat, to survive, to have sex, to reproduce, to ensure the perpetuation of our own genes.

Fighting, drinking, gambling, wanton pillage; morality is ephemeral and in another cultural milieu these activities might be looked on with undiluted admiration. Being nice to each other is just a current fad, and under the skin we are red in tooth and claw and other more sensitive body parts.

One of the great and unabashedly atavistic male pleasures is wiping another guy's eye — that is, taking his girl — preferably in public; telling your mates about it later, though an exquisite joy in its own right, is but the icing on the cake. Admit it lads; doesn't it feel good? It's a way of staking out our ground, showing how tough and hard we are.

And Dr Fitzpiers, the country GP from Thomas Hardy's *The Woodlanders*, may therefore have been an unwitting role model for many of us, and perhaps a subliminal reason for us becoming doctors in the first place. Poor old horny-handed redneck Giles Winterborne is in love with college-educated-beyond-her-station Grace Melbury, his employer's daughter, in what seems a most congenial arrangement. She seems fond of him also, though in a patronising puppy-dog kind of way, until Fitzpiers comes into town, a combination of cynicism and arrogance that she finds both repellent and irresistible. As the saying goes: good girls, bad boys, even badder docs, though nowadays Fitzpiers would be struck off quicker than you can say Jude the Obscure.

And what's love got to do with it, Fitzpiers might have said as he rushed off to a tryst with the lady of the manor, having just enjoyed Suke Damson's more pastoral and toothy charms.

And we have other tendencies that might be frowned on, but are integral parts of our drive to achieve and prosper. When I was a poor doctor, I hated rich doctors. I hated their nice suits and their silk ties and their big shiny cars and their complacency and their arrogance and their tennis clubs and the way they didn't sweat much.

And when I became a rich doc — rich relative to my previous poverty, I mean — I turned right around and started hating poor docs, hating their grubby suits, their beat up old cars, and especially their idealism and enthusiasm. Greed and begrudgery, what would we do without them?

It's the classic Irish success story.

Footnote; dedicated to my friend Kieran Connolly, my own role-model (which is why I've turned out so well).

Beauty of the drug rep

GP 20 March 2015

Farrell's First Law (immutable); in any photograph of any medical meeting, the good-looking ones are always the drug reps.

The heart never gets to take a break. Unlike our brain, liver or kidneys, which can nod off to sleep now and then, and nobody will notice, our heart has to keep going non-stop, not even taking five minutes for a cup of coffee and a big doughnut or to nip out the back for a quick smoke. And it is always vulnerable.

Our eyes met, smouldering. This is a Moment, I thought; stay with it, relish every second, this Moment of trumpets and flowers and bright mornings and rich beds and birds singing and blue skies, a Moment even worth tweeting about. Apropos of nothing, I hadn't been laid in a really long time; soft flesh and my hot Spanish blood, you would need a prostate to really understand.

Her cheekbones were so high, they must have needed oxygen tanks. Beauty may be only skin deep, but that's deep enough for me. I'm superficial myself, so I quite understood; between the two of us there was just enough for a shallow pond. And as Friedrich Holderlin observed in Socrates and Alcibiades, 'The wise, in the end/Must always bow to the beautiful.'

'For I would ride with you upon the wind,' I wanted to say to her, 'run on the top of the dishevelled tide, and dance upon the mountains like a flame.'

Yet beauty can be as dangerous as fire. What use are dreams if they can't be shattered? What use is a heart if it can't be broken? When you light a candle, you also cast a shadow.

She looked at me and said: 'Can I interest you in our new non-steroidal anti-inflammatory?'

Chapter 3

Birth and family

You can choose your friends, but you're stuck with your relations; I learned this from an early age. We had a gargantuan family circle, in a constant dynamic state, new babies added on even as we lost older clumsier ones through frequent barnyard accidents.

In particular I had a large number of religiously fanatical aunties; this might be considered a bad thing, but to paraphrase the eminent psychiatrist Dr Frasier Crane, if you can't laugh at your family, what good are they?

No laughing matter?

BMJ 27 May 1995

It was the usual labour ward pandemonium: a slow breech delivery; a multiparous woman with her feet up in stirrups; an exasperated nurse holding her hand; and blood, sweat, tears, liquor, meconium, and other less salubrious body fluids flying everywhere.

My colleague was a tall, handsome, effortlessly charming Australian. We were waiting at the business end; we had been very concerned about fetal distress, and had almost reached panic level, but the clinical picture had suddenly improved, and the crisis seemed to be over. We had both heaved a huge sigh of relief and now we could just about see the breech coming down.

'Can you see my baby yet?' cried the woman to the nurse.

'No,' she replied soothingly, 'but doctor can.'

'Don't worry,' said my friend encouragingly, with what he obviously considered to be a disarming smile, 'I can see baby coming; she's got a lovely little bottom;' he paused and winked at me, 'just like you, ma'am.' If it hadn't been for the stirrups she would have kicked him.

This almost true story, funny at the time, doesn't seem so amusing now, but we all know even worse tales, all too upsetting even to consider putting down in print; there seems to be no such thing as a taboo subject. The more exquisite the agony, the more bleak the outcome, the more callous the humour becomes. The greater the human calamity, the later the hour, and the more exhausted and inexperienced the doctors, the more blithe the relish with which the tale is told.

But why should such a bizarre trait persist in what is supposed to be a 'caring profession'? Humour is surely one of the strangest aspects of the human condition. What purpose does it have? What genetic drive has led to its perpetuation in our genome? There must be some survival value in being able to look on the funny side, humour being a plant that thrives in adversity.

In medicine we daily perform a balancing act between normality on one side and disaster on the other and one of the ways we cope with the frequent lurches into tragedy is to disarm it by reducing it to an object of derision. Comedy is a way of demystifying those things we fear and don't understand. We can't be frightened of something we have just made ridiculous. After all, comedy and tragedy are so far apart that, if certain unconventional theories about the structure of the universe are true, they are practically next door to each other.

Medical humour helps us to bear the unbearable. Each man mourns in his own way; in the caring nineties, if it's all right for a grown man to cry, it should be all right for him to laugh as well.

Give the kid a chance

GP 4 November 2010

Names can be tricky; Terry Pratchett described one set of devout but confused parents who got mixed up between the virtues and the seven deadly sins, all of which resulted in their children being called Faith, Hope, and Bestiality. And just to show how misleading a label can be, Bestiality Carter was actually very kind to animals.

'How old is baby?' I asked. I used the non-gender-specific noun because I didn't know whether it was a boy or girl, and family doctors are supposed to know this kind of stuff. Usually there are clues, boys in blue, girls in pink, but this baby was swaddled in neutral and uninformative butterfly yellow. But time reveals all, and the experienced GP is patient, yet always alert and watchful for even the most subtle intimation.

'She's two weeks today,' said mother proudly, solving the mystery.

'Isn't she a beautiful little girlie, what are you calling her?', I asked, compensating for my previous obfuscation with a spatter of personal pronouns, 'Mary-Kate would be nice, after her granny on her father's side, the one who punched Florence Nightingale during the Crimean War.'

'No, that's much too old-fashioned, I wanted something new and different,' she said.

'Like Kylie or Britney,' I suggested (I am still pretty hip, you see, and right in touch with 'yoof' culture).

'No, far too common,' she said. 'I heard a lovely name recently, so we are going to call her - Cialis.'

There was a long silence, punctuated only by the clunky sound of my jaw hitting the floor. It was none of my business really, but sometimes a doctor's duties extend far beyond the narrow church of medicine, so I felt obliged to intervene.

'Ci-a-lis,' I said, pronouncing it extremely slowly, trying to give her a hint that there was major drawback here. 'Your husband's suggestion, I presume?'

'Yes,' she said happily. 'I think he got it from one of his friends. It sounds so graceful and feminine, doesn't it, like a swallow's flight, and there won't be any other girls with that name.'

'You can be sure about that,' I confirmed

Footnote; Cialis is a similar medication to Viagra, used for the same romantic purpose.

Auntz

GP 20 August 2009

My aunties Josie and Mary had lived together for generations in amicably combative spinsterhood. Auntie Mary was lively and jolly, Auntie Josie was a whiny old torture. Of course, life not being fair, Auntie Mary died first.

The funeral was Auntie Josie's big day; she was the chief mourner, the team captain, and she played the role with gusto, flogging it mercilessly, born to wear the black, metaphorically shouting 'It's all about Me! Me! Me!'

Tradition would have dictated that the deceased only be kept one night in the house, and then one night in the church, but Auntie Josie wanted the whole hog, such was her inconsolable grief and unadulterated desire for attention, so Auntie Mary was waked at home for both nights.

I sat up the first night of the wake with sundry uncles and cousins, telling funny stories about Auntie Mary, of which there were plenty, Auntie Josie all the while hovering in the background checking that the corpse wasn't moving.

However, come the second night, when a night's sleep might also have been considered traditional, Auntie Josie, being the star of the show, insisted on staying up again and in the deep of the night I received a panicky phone-call from my brother. Auntie Josie, he said, had 'took out' and I was to come out and give her something, me being a doctor and all. Had I been older and more worldly-wise I'd have declined the honour, but I was young and easily manipulated.

When I arrived Auntie Josie was rampaging around the room, my brother, aunties and cousins cowering in the corner. I calmed Auntie Josie down; Auntie Mary was not moving, I assured her and yes, she really was in the bosom of Abraham and not just playing a funny trick.

But as I had an audience, and lay people have nothing but contempt for talking cures, To Show How Much I Care, and to be seen to be doing something, I gave Auntie Josie a paracetamol, a placebo I reckoned would not interrupt the grieving process too much.

The next day, Auntie Josie collapsed in front of the church, in a way only a really fit person could collapse, in stages, like a dying (if rather overweight) swan.

'What did you give her?' hissed my brother accusingly.

The Hunting of the Snark

GP 5 Feb 2009

'In the midst of the thing he was trying to say/In the midst of his laughter and glee/He had slowly and silently faded away/For the Snark was a Boojum, you see.'

Lewis Carroll's outre poem about an unlikely crew in search of an impossible creature has long mystified scholars. What was the intended allegory, what was a snark, what was a boojum? Well, my long and bitter life experience has suggested one plausible interpretation; the snark, I conjecture, is a metaphor for unrealistic expectations, and a boojum when those expectations get busted.

As a lad I had two elderly aunties, Josie and Mary, spinsters who lived together. On one occasion Mary had to be admitted to hospital, and my brother Tommy, who was like Mother Teresa without the cool white gear and the expensive PR, undertook to drive Josie to the hospital each night to visit Mary.

One night, Tommy was busy and asked if I would help out. 'Like I don't have a life,' I said, but because I am sometimes a good person, I agreed to substitute, strictly for one night only.

But the substitution was not acceptable to Mary, and I was forced to endure a haemorrhage of whinging and moaning all the way to the hospital, 'Tommy Farrell let me down, I'll never depend on him again, who does he think he is etc..,' My brother had set up the expectation, and reaped the unrelenting ingratitude of a sad and bitter old woman.

During the Troubles there were frequent bomb attacks on the local army barracks, thoughtfully situated in the village square. After one bomb, I called to check on the

47

Maguires, an elderly couple living on the square. It was really just a social visit, as I was passing by, but while there I checked their blood pressure, the medical equivalent of kicking for touch, making it look like we are actually doing something.

It was nothing heroic, I know, just a small random act of kindness, but a few days later, there was another bomb on the square. I'd been off, so when I arrived back I asked my partner about casualties.

'None,' he said, 'But the Maguires called, very upset they were, after waiting up all night to have their blood pressure taken.'

The snark had become a boojum.

Auntz again

BMJ 9 December 2000

Auntie Josie had situational dementia. A large lady, she came to live with us after her third stroke, and as my parents were dead she immediately assumed responsibility for my spiritual welfare.

All week she would sit cackling maniacally by the fire, immovable in voluminous black skirts, but come Sunday morning a miracle would occur. She would arise like a massive billowing dark Lazarus, filled with a fanatical zeal to ensure that I attended church. Her Christianity was of that peculiarly Northern Ireland brand: whenever two or three are gathered together in my name some other poor bastard is going to get a good kicking. Salmon Rushdie and I, we understand fatwas.

So from 8 am Auntie Josie would be tugging at my bedclothes with surprising strength and tenacity for someone who midweek couldn't lift a teacup. By the time of the last mass, if I was still in situ, she'd be spinning around in a frenzy.

I tolerated this ritual as a kind of tough love, because Auntie Josie had reason to be fond of me. Another auntie, Auntie Beattie (not a blood relation), was given to boasting about her big babies; all eight were over 10 pounds at birth. This was perceived as a jibe at the lack of fecundity of my blood aunts, none of whom had children, only a few of whom were married, and all of whom were virgins. It's impossible to have sex while kneeling in church, which for my aunts was a 24-hour commitment.

One day at dinner, Auntie Beattie was telling everybody for the cajillionth time how the obstetrician said, 'You've done it again, Mrs Boyle,' when she delivered her 10th baby, apparently as big as a hippo.

But by this time, I had become a doctor and had rocketed from being an insignificant guttersnipe to the next best thing to the Pope.

'There's a bit of diabetes in your family, isn't there?' I inquired, in the style of Emile Zola. 'Could be why all your babies were such whoppers; *j'accuse*!!'

There was immediate uproar; my blood aunties were jumping up and down with excitement, while Auntie Beattie was incandescent with outrage that these highlights of an otherwise implacably mundane life could be so glibly dismissed as merely the consequence of a family delicacy.

Order was eventually restored by the old 'I've got a gun' trick, but the seed of doubt had been planted, and we never heard those gargantuan baby stories ever again.

Wii-habilitation

BMJ 25 March 2009

In Ireland we have an ancient law that the more obnoxious a relative, the more likely they are to gravitate towards your hearth. My many siblings were at first quite
willing to shoulder their fair share of the burden, but they
mysteriously developed a serious and disfiguring infectious disease just as Auntie Josie's massive orbit was
about to degrade into devastating planetfall.

Auntie Josie's disposition was not kindly. Her religious
begrudgery, in that great tradition stretching from Tor-
quemada to the Taliban, decreed that not only was the
glass half empty, some other greedy bastard had already
drunk the best of it. When my little Gracie was born, and
I presented her to Auntie Josie, I expected at least a few
bills and coos. 'Little girls were born to suffer,' she said.

And at Christmas she would observe, 'Christmas is a sad
time, very sad,' for an encore describing, in lurid detail,
with added sound effects, her latest revolting bowel complaint. Take all the fun in the world and get rid of it, that's
how much fun she was, maybe the reason there are no
jolly Christmas songs about elderly aunts.

But even in winter, the cold isn't always bitter and not
every day is cruel, and something wonderful happened
last Christmas Eve, on that most magical night of the
year.

I woke in the early hours, disturbed by an unfamiliar
sound. It sounded like . . . chuckling, which slowly increased in volume and pitch until peals of girlish laughter
were ringing in the air like silver bells. I slipped on the
pyjamas Santa inexplicably brings every year, crept
downstairs, and peeped into the living room, where I be-
held a remarkable sight.

Auntie Josie was hippety-hopping up and down on the Wii, Santa's present for my daughter Gracie. Encouraged by the onscreen homunculus, she spun and pirouetted like a gazelle; for a woman whose only usual activity had been to squat toad-like in front of the fire, this was an unprecedented demonstration of gymnastic dexterity. And the true miracle of Christmas: she looked happy. Like the ranks of Tuscany, I could 'scarce forbear to cheer,' especially with the prospect of an entertaining flatline. What better way to go, I mused, than among family who love you, or can barely tolerate you.

Since then not only have her balance, posture, and mobility improved, but her demeanour has also moderated.

This Damascene epiphany is anecdotal evidence only, but imagine a Wii for every nursing home, every house with a granny, and every couch potato and the incalculable possibilities in rehabilitation and restoring mobility and general jollification. Of course, once the Wii is medicalised we'll need health and safety assessments, training courses, tutors, diplomas, degrees, professors, academic processions, but it will be worth the pain.

If the Wii can render my Auntie Josie slightly less homicidal, it can do anything.

She didn't actually try to stab me the next day. At the Farrell family Christmas, that's what we call a result.

Tea?

British Journal of General Practice May 2000

When I was a lad we had lots of aunties, all of them fanatically devout. On one occasion, my Auntie Susie returned from pilgrimage and brought back, as A Present From Religious-19th centuryVille, a little three-legged tea-stand. In rural Ireland, most of our lives were spent in the kitchen and the present was, accordingly, displayed there to all the family, plus assembled hangers-on, plus other aunties. We had a colossal family circle that was in a constant dynamic equilibrium: people coming, people going, babies being born, grannies dying, young people emigrating or losing body parts in farm accidents.

The little tea-stand received general approval, even from the other aunts, who were usually viciously critical about everything; it was a default option, as my aunts were committed Luddites. Perhaps they were seduced by the picture on the base of St. Luke removing a sebaceous cyst from the Good Samaritan's armpit, and also the tea-stand had irrefutable qualities of both practicality (the table cloth and table would not be singed), and of presentation (the teapot would at last have its rightful place at the top of the table, and now especially set upon a throne which originated in Religious-19thcenturyVille).

The friends, relatives, and aunts accordingly assembled in their accustomed places around the kitchen table, hundreds of them to my child's eye, and the table appeared as big as a football field, which is not as great an exaggeration as you might think, as in those days football pitches were rather small and distressingly full of cows and cow dung. And then someone had an idea which seemed appropriate, if devastatingly lacking in originality: 'Let's have a cup of tea'.

Our teapot held about ten gallons and took three people to carry. Despite this size it had a seemingly magical quality in that it never ran out, no matter how thirsty the residents, no matter how many visitors might arrive at the last moment, aching for succour; there was always enough tea in that teapot, and so there was a vague ceremonial air as it was set upon the little tea-stand, a bit like you British guys getting knighted, I reckon.

For one brief glorious moment it perched there, a moment just long enough to catch a glint of the sun's rays through the kitchen window, a golden moment redolent of Druids and Winter Solstices and New-age hippies and meticulously plotted prehistoric maths and fleetingly sunlit tombs and virgins being sacrificed. Then the laws of physics, which had briefly nodded off, perhaps enchanted by the earth-power, reasserted themselves and realised that the whole structure was about as unstable as a sack of plutonium being flogged to Japan by Sellafield.

One of the legs of the tea-stand buckled and the teapot toppled over, exploding onto the table. A tidal wave of hot tea surged across the table and down onto the laps of those clustered closest around it; as my aunties were most senior in the hierarchy, they always had pride of place sitting in close to the table, the rest of us palely loitering round the door and leaning on the side-board. This usually meant they had first choice of whatever delicacy was on offer, invariably fresh bread and scones, and a better vantage position to dominate whatever bitter and divisive family argument was in progress, but on this day it proved to be an unlucky choice.

Boy, it was funny — those aunts could move quick when they wanted to; pain is a great motivator.

Especially when it's your own.

Blue blood

BMJ 3 December 2008

As a baby I was of royal blood, closely related to the Dauphin - close enough, like Sarah Palin, to see the Russian royal family from my house. Unfortunately, on the day I was presented to the adoring masses the ceremony was hijacked by the Evil Fairy, who stole me from a life of Parisian splendour and decadence and for good measure chucked in the vices of Greed, Lust, Envy, Gluttony, Sarcasm, and, finally, just to prove that the devil has all the best jokes, Bestiality.

Fortunately, just before I was spirited away to rural Ireland, the Good Fairy turned up. Unfortunately, because she was so late (apparently Cinderella had needed emergency contraception and was too thick to realise that it was available from any pharmacy), she couldn't restore my rightful place among the crowned heads of Europe, nor were there any other decent presents handy. The only gift she had left was Sloth, which she reckoned would protect me from the worst excesses of the other vices, all of which need a bit of enthusiasm.

Thanks for nothing, lady, I might have said, now sod off back to your gingerbread cottage.

Which explains why I have always been seriously lazy and chose general practice as a vocation. Dressing in tweeds, smoking a pipe, walking the dog, sitting back in a comfortable chair listening to people drone on and on, idly tootling down country roads gazing speculatively at the sheep: it was the perfect career for me.

But not anymore, because family doctors are getting ever busier, partly because of a mushrooming bureaucracy and partly the result of the inexorable advance of scientific knowledge, which sometimes trickles down eventually to us. For example, 15 years ago patients with atrial fibrillation were put on digoxin, and that was more or less the end of it; now they need warfarin, with all the associated supervision it demands.

And with every advance it's not as if something drops off the back of the bus to compensate. We can't stop seeing kids with upper respiratory tract infections, varicose veins still need to be referred, and cardiac risk factors still need to be modified. The workload is ever expanding.

I expressed my frustration to my Auntie Mamie.

'C'est la vie, your majesty,' she sympathised.

Chapter 4
The art of medicine

Other medical disciplines are fortunate. They are more predictable and can apply more scientific rigour; their maps are complete, easier to plot. General practice, by contrast, is the great unknown. We stand on the cusp of the beyond; science takes us only so far, then the maps stop in the grey areas of intuition, imagination and feelings, here be dragons.

Lurching from heart-breaking tragedy to high farce, we are the Renaissance men and women of medicine; our art is intangible and almost impossible to pigeon-hole. Anything can walk through our door; whatever it is, we have to handle it.

There is more to a surgery than bricks and mortar, more to a doctor's office than just a desk and an examination couch. It's a place of comfort and caring, a place where you will always be listened to, where someone, somehow will always try to make you feel better.

Stand outside the health centre for a moment, and if you scrunch up your eyes a little, and use your imagination, you can almost picture it as a medieval castle, a sanctuary defending your people against all plagues and evils; a symbol that the world can be kind and gentle.

And for our part, it feels good to be needed, no matter how humble the service we provide. We stand between the candle and the darkness, and though the battle cannot be won maybe today will bring a small victory.

During every surgery there is something to be won; we always have options, though those options may really,

really suck. What may seem trivial and banal to the out-side and uninformed observer, may have deeper, life-changing significance.

As Patrick Kavanagh observed, 'Till Homer's ghost came whispering to my mind/He said: I made The Iliad from such/A local row. Gods make their own im-portance.'

Deeply moving

BMJ 13 October 2001

If a tree falls in the forest and no one is there to hear, does it make a sound?

One of a doctor's unwritten roles is just to be there, to be a witness, a witness to pain and suffering, to grief and loss, to moments of great joy and great sorrow, but most of all a witness to body fluids.

Mrs Keogh arrived in the surgery in what P G Wode-house would have called a dignified procession of one. 'What do you think of that, doctor?' she asked, burping open the Tupperware container.

There followed a long, contemplative, and unexpectedly companionable silence; a golden, serene moment, a time for pause and quiet reflection, a time to stop and smell the flowers in a world that rushes ever faster. As the air grew steamy around us I could see little motes of dust sparkling in a stray gleam of sunlight through the win-dow and hear far away in the distance a small aeroplane purring over the meadows. The surgery had the spiritual ambience of a monastery chapel, and if C S Lewis and J R R Tolkien had walked in twittering gently on about morality and suspiciously androgynous fairies, I would-n't have been surprised.

Eventually, and not without some feeling of loss, I surfaced. 'That is a very impressive bowel motion, ma'am,' I said slowly, 'a very impressive bowel motion indeed, the very opposite of jejune, the apotheosis of the gold bar; an unforgettable bouquet, lines as sleek as a thoroughbred racehorse, and a colour deep and mysterious as a Conrad novel. If it could talk it would have the rich, fruity timbre of Anthony Hopkins, and it would tell us of a digestive system in excellent, nay, in exquisite shape, bespeaking a diet rich in all the fine things of this goodly earth. If this were the Olympics, we could hang the medal round its finely tapered neck right now.'

But Mrs Keogh had yet another surprise for me. 'It's not mine, it's my husband's,' she said, her voice soft with tenderness. 'Isn't it a beauty?'

Some married couples are just a little too intimate, I thought; 'Love sees not with the eyes but with the mind/And thus is winged Cupid ever painted blind.'

'If you love something, let it go,' I paraphrased solemnly, 'If it loves you, it will come back; if it gets flushed down the toilet, you don't want it.

Norm must go

BMJ 1 December 2005

Dysorganophilia (Farrell's syndrome): excessive affection for an abnormal body part.

When I was a lad I had a papilloma on my left upper arm, and had no need of thumb-sucking or a security blanket; I had Bob to twiddle, and we went everywhere together.

'Isn't he a gorgeous little thing?' girlfriends would say, admiring the elegant stalk, the smooth bulbous head, but as I grew older, more mature and sophisticated, and conscious of the importance of physical perfection, I became embarrassed by Bob. Even on nudist beaches, where I was unashamed to let everything else hang out, I would hide Bob with a bandage.

Eventually I decided Bob had to go.

The razor felt cold, ice against my skin. And a drop of blood welled up like a last tear—had I heard a sad little sigh? I left Bob dead and with his head I went galumphing back to the world of normal people.

But years later, I found I was not alone.

Joe refused to have Norm removed, as he had become rather inappropriately fond of his hydrocoele. As I had worn the T shirt, I could empathise; Norm was cheaper and less troublesome than a pet, didn't leave a mess, didn't need a licence, didn't need to be taken for walks.

Every so often, when Norm became so large that Joe required an extra seat on the bus he would let me drain off a few gallons, but it was a procedure that caused him considerable distress.

'Ah, look at the poor wee thing, don't be taking too much now,' he would say. 'No more, no more, for God's sake hasn't he suffered enough?'

'There, there,' I would say, as counselling is so important; sometimes I think I Care Too Much.

Joe would then stand shaking himself for a few moments, getting used to his altered centre of gravity. His mood would also be altered, but as the weeks passed and the implacable forces of physiology forced vibrant life-affirming fluids back into the temporarily flaccid Norm, Joe would regain his jaunty good humour.

'And Norm gives my girlfriends such a scare,' he said, grinning evilly.

'I don't know about your girlfriends,' I said, like the Iron Duke reviewing his troops before Waterloo, 'but by God, he scares me.'

Footnote: A papilloma is a little squishy skin lump; a hydrocoele is a fluid-filled cyst on the testicles.

Great Toe of this Assembly

BMJ 9 February 2006

Referring to yourself in the third person usually signifies an unpleasantly inflated ego—for example, 'The Lady's not for turning.' But I can do better, with echoes of the politically incorrect 'Liver in ward 3.'

It was a cold winter's night, and the wind was moaning through the eaves like a patient having an in-grown toe-nail removed who has been given too little local anaesthetic (come on, haven't we all done it?), the kind of night when doctors huddle a little closer to the fire, like a blob of phlegm on the uvula.

Then, the phone call.

'What about The Toe?' said a voice, and that was all it said.

I was lost in the ambiguity.

'What about The Toe?' I repeated it softly to myself, a question leading only to more questions. Whose toe? Why are we here? What was wrong with The Toe to begin with?

Yet there was information to be gleaned: an implacable self-confidence, certainty that his voice would be instantly recognised, and that his Toe was unforgettable, contempt for Galileo and Copernicus and all those who had endured persecution in search of scientific truth. The earth doesn't revolve around the sun, everything revolves around me. Me, me, I am the Great Panjandrum.

I wished, once again, that Sigmund Freud was still around to help; note the subject's terse and precise language, he would say.

'How anal of you to notice,' I would reply.

'Oh, everything's anal to you,' he would scoff. '

'Why, does it remind you of your mummy?' I would retort.

'You speak the truth, my young Oedipus,' he would say. 'We must investigate.'

When I arrived at the farm, everything was quiet, apart from the slavering guard dog, which, unusually, had three heads.

A hawthorn grew in the centre of the yard, which made turning awkward. It hadn't been chopped down, as the hawthorn had a reputation as a faery tree, so I resisted the temptation to drive over it.

The Toe was reclining regally on a velvet cushion. 'Great Toe of this assembly,' I said, giving it a respectful little massage and some antibiotics (as is traditional in the country) and advising it to rest.

The owner regarded me with satisfaction.

'Look on The Toe, ye mighty,' he said, 'and despair.'

Medical conferences/wildlife documentaries

GP 1 December 2015

It must be tough being a penguin; not only are you being constantly harassed by film crews, who love the fact that you can't fly away, but Morgan Freeman is always popping up from behind an iceberg and global warming is increasingly degrading your breeding grounds and food supplies.

And my proposal to ease the impact of global warming will make it even tougher; move the polar bears to the Antarctic, where there'll be plenty of penguins for them to eat (and they can't fly away). I've written to David Attenborough and expect the great man to be in touch shortly.

I do love the BBC wildlife documentaries, but the postscripts which show the lengths they go to film them are equally arresting.

So often it seems that, after months of squatting in sweaty bug-infested squalor, they always seem to get the footage only on the very last day. Perhaps it would be much more efficient and economical if all fieldwork and shoots should be restricted to a single day (in effect, the very last day)

This has medical implications also. I enjoy conferences; being lectured by specialists who know nothing about the realities of general practice is like watching Fox News, it's always satisfying to have your prejudices confirmed.

But every conference should have a fake last lecture, because the real last lecture is always given by a second-rater and the attendance is always threadbare - the delegates having already signed in for the PGE credits and sneaked off early to catch an early train or have a few beers and a booty call.

As the audience progressively dwindled at one conference I attended, no-one even bothering to tweet, it got more and more embarrassing for those left behind, and ever harder to slip out the back unnoticed; but the momentum was unstoppable, until by the end it was just me and the lecturer in the vast, echoing auditorium (and the janitor, standing impatiently at the sidelines).

'Any questions?' asked the lecturer, with rather desperate enthusiasm.

'I have one; are you nearly finished?' said the janitor.

'Did you understand the main point?' the lecturer, this time directing the question directly to me, obviously anxious for feedback.

'Yes,' I said. 'Never, ever, get stuck with the last lecture.'

Nemesis

BMJ 29 September 2010

It seemed to taunt me: 'I am the eternal abscess. I have been your companion through the ages, adorning both knight and burgher, proud and red and ripe and rampant. Shakespeare immortalised me as 'imposthume.' But the sin of Hubris is always punished by Nemesis, just back from a long weekend with Sappho in Lesbos.

'I think we'd better lance this,' I'd said, although this was just foreplay, because our nurse was the true connoisseur.

'Things growing are not ripe until their season,' she murmured, half to herself, eyeing it keenly, fondling it a bit (a bit too much, I reckon; certainly more than was entirely decent), like Ernest and Julio Gallo checking out their grapes. 'It will be pointing in, I would estimate,' she mused, 'about three days.'

And sure enough, three days later, 'Macbeth is ripe for picking,' she said, purring with anticipation, her lips moist and wanton and come hither. The vorpal blade went snicker-snack, and the laudable pus came spurting out, like wandering water gushing from the hills above Glencar, after which we felt compelled, for some inexplicable reason, to nip out the back for a languorous smoke.

But this unusual consummation was only the prologue; she also took extreme offence at any pus that remained unexpressed, so she returned to combat, put Wagner's *Ride of the Valkyries* on the CD player, and squeezed and squeezed like her life depended on it. As the abscess was out of the patient's eye-line, she gave a running commentary to keep the patient informed and the rest of us entertained.

'You should see the stuff coming out of it now, what a rich and glorious colour; earth has not anything to show more fair; what a vibrant and unforgettable bouquet; it's amazing; it's incredible; just one more squeeze; don't worry, we're nearly finished now; just the last wee bit; gosh, can you believe it, there's loads more, buckets and buckets of it, where is it all coming from? Ah, look, there's another abscess; that one's not ready yet: you'll have to come back next week.'

And then, aside to the audience, 'Always leave 'em begging for more.'

Relationships can be toxic

BMJ 19 January 2002

Laurel: 'What's for supper, Ollie?'

Hardy: 'Fries and beans, Stanley.'

Laurel: 'Gee, Ollie, you sure know how to plan a meal.'

Laurel innocently fuels Hardy's conceit, and the boys are much too contented. They have committed the sin of hubris and you know disaster is about to befall them. With the right partner either Laurel or Hardy might have gone far, but their mutual dependency feeds their worst qualities and constantly places them in impossible situations, like trying to carry a piano across a rope bridge between two alpine cliffs with a gorilla in the middle.

Forget viruses, bacteria, trauma, cigarettes, radioactivity—what screws most people up is relationships, with other people mostly.

I'd like to quote myself: 'If general practitioners have any specialty it is the individual.' But once it goes beyond one man and becomes a man and a woman, or two men, or two women, or one more woman going nowhere just for show, with the church maybe getting into bed beside them to complete the brew, no understanding is possible.

If it was only as simple as drug interactions. My pharmacist can call me and say, 'That guy you prescribed aspirin for, he's on warfarin, and you wanted him to have verapamil, but he's already on digoxin.' And I can reply, 'Thanks, pal, you take over his medical management, and I'll flog him some cheap aftershave.'

But there is no predictability to relationships, no database to allow any kind of rational forecast; we throw our balls up in the air and they come down in a totally random manner. Two beautiful and gentle people can produce plutonium, two obnoxious and dysfunctional people can sing as sweetly as a linnet.

Trying to help in any way is fraught with pearls. Non-directional counselling and a sympathetic ear are usually the most we can offer. Anything more interventionist invites retaliation; no longer a soothing escape valve, we have become part of the problem.

Joe had a Medical Oedipus Complex; he wanted to sleep with his mother and kill his doctor.

'I'm angry with my wife and my kids and my boss,' he said, 'but most of all, doctor, I'm angry with you.'

Natural? No thanks

BMJ 28 April 2005

'I don't want any drugs,' she said, 'I'd like something natural.'

The term 'natural' is a broad and much-abused church. In terms of Things GPs Don't Like To Hear, it's right up there with 'He's pulling at his ears.' It refers to the material world and to those phenomena that function independently of humans, but somewhere along the line, like 'detox' and 'herbal,' it became hijacked by the marketing men into a Sunday feature magazine bourgeois conceit: shampoos with 'natural' spices, skin creams with miraculously anti-ageing 'natural' herbs, 'natural' products evangelically and uncritically fêted as remedies for every conceivable complaint, with attractive exotic names like black hellebore, ginkgo biloba.

It's even better if they come from the rain forest—endangered rainforest is best, especially if it has evening primrose oil in it.

In the latter mode 'natural' really means 'completely untested, bugger all use, but probably safe and nicely expensive and a good earner for some crafty sod.' Strangely, people who have to live in the rain forest would prefer to have antibiotics and vaccines and maybe some anti-fungal creams for those eternally sweaty arm-pits and groins.

Opium is natural, as is phlegm, and vomiting and diar-rhoea. If we left it up to nature, life would be nasty, brut-ish, and short; as hunter-gatherers we rarely lived to be 40, infant mortality was at least 250 per 1000 births, and half of us were dead by 5 years of age.

On the positive side of this pre-Raphaelite fairy tale ex-istence, there were no worries about the side-effects of hormone replacement therapy, because the menopause was nature's way of telling us we were mouldy and ob-solete and to make room for the young and good-looking. Lifestyle changes were not an issue because we didn't live long enough to get cancers and heart disease (we could have smoked our brains out in those days, no prob-lem).

Nature is not cuddly and benevolent; it is cold, unfeeling and indifferent, and surrenders its charms grudgingly; any concessions have been wrested from it only by thou-sands of years of painstaking effort laced with occasional flashes of genius, often in the face of prejudice and per-secution, thumbscrews, and iron maidens.

'Well,' I replied, 'we could just do nothing and let you die; it doesn't come any more natural than that.'

Treasure those complaints

GP 10 October 2012

Complaints are precious, I read somewhere; we should hoard them like jewels, for only through complaints do we realise how our services are deficient and how to cor-rect the deficiency.

Compliments, by contrast, are dangerous, because they are less likely to be true than complaints, encourage complacency, and may be manipulative.

Well, blow that for a game of soldiers, I say.

We put up a complaints box and all we got was a scrawl of obscene graffiti implying that my partner had a big butt (and there's nothing we can do about that, he's stuck with it).

'Before I start,' the patient said, 'I would like to say how much I admire your achievements.'

'Thanks,' I said.

'Not yours in particular, I mean,' he continued. 'The whole scientific medical thing.'

'On behalf of the whole medical community,' I said, 'I accept your thanks, it really means a lot to us that you recognise the sacrifices of Galileo, the brilliance of Pasteur, the perspicacity of Fleming, the way in which knowledge has been gleaned, often in the face of persecution and superstition. I'll organise a press release for the BBC. They make such a fuss about the Nobel Prize, but this is much more important and gratifying.'

'However,' he said. 'There is one thing that I'm not happy about.'

'Contrary to expectations,' I said, 'my job is not to make you happy. Happiness is ephemeral, way beyond my humble remit.'

'The waiting room is not restful and relaxing,' he said. 'The chairs are uncomfortable, there's no TV or wi-fi and the magazines are all gossipy tabloids. Why don't you have *The Economist*?'

'Oooh,' I said, rather impressed.

'The posters on the walls are out of date,' he said. 'And the walls are painted a nauseating greenish colour.'

'You may be under a misapprehension,' I explained. 'The waiting room is not supposed to be a garden of delights, it's for waiting. You may also have noticed the absence of lace cloths and wine-buckets; this ain't no whorehouse parlour.'

'You aren't taking me seriously,' he said, 'Can I see another doctor?'

'Of course,' I said, always ready to help, 'Just take a seat in the waiting room.'

Small is Beautiful

BMJ 22 March 1997

My home village, Rostrevor, lies between the Mourne Mountains and Carlingford Lough, but it's not an uncomfortable perch, as if the mountains don't like us and are slowly pushing us into the sea. We get on better than that with our native soil; the Mournes are protective, and Rostrevor nestles under their armpit as snugly as a wee mouse in a corn-stack. This is not entirely fanciful; the Mournes deflect the worst snows and the sea breezes ameliorate the worst frosts, and during the Great Hunger, Rostrevor was untouched by typhoid fever, although the potato blight did hit us hard.

A Canadian visitor was unimpressed.

'Heck,' he said, 'You call those little things mountains? The Rockies are ten times the size.'

'Oh, like you built them yourself, did you?' I retorted, for I like the Mournes just the way they are; accessible and not too rugged, so that you can climb them without Sherpas, drop a bottle of stout in a mountain stream, and when just cool enough share it with the skylarks and the ravens before taking out a big cigar and sending smoke rings floating gracefully down the breeze.

Bigness is not a virtue; there is a defining quality to small things, like a Seurat masterpiece, where omission of even one dot can lose an eye, a smile, even a mood, and irredeemably change the nature of the whole picture.

A geneticist surveyed 6000 people to find the true sources of happiness. 'Find the small things that give a little high.' he advised, 'a good meal, working in the garden, time with friends. Sprinkle your life with them, and they will leave you happier than the grand achievement that lasts for only a while.'

I could add; the rim of froth on your upper lip after a draught of Guinness; that first smoke after good sex; the coda to Beethoven's Ninth Symphony.

But small things can be a bugger, like the lad who complained of having sweaty feet. He wasn't exaggerating, and the room was filled with a fruity odour, almost pleasant if its origin had been unknown. This was, he surmised, stopping him getting a girlfriend. But I probed deeper, and found he was a Garth Brooks fan, and so technically undateable, be his feet as fragrant as Mary Archer's.

So as well as medical advice, I loaned him some James Brown tapes and when he returned both his sweaty feet and his social life had greatly improved. Boy meets girl, boy has sweaty feet, boy goes to doctor, boy gets girl.

It's the classic Irish love story.

My (real) role-model

GP 4 December 2017

'Ah, the fall of the leaf,' said my senior colleague happily, as we drove slowly down the boreen. 'There is still magic in the world.'

He had been retired for many years but enjoyed accompanying me on house calls. He'd looked after our patients for over fifty years, battling ceaselessly through the dark times of the Troubles, bearing unfailing witness to the joys and sorrows of generations, and I always felt very fortunate to be accompanied by his wisdom and knowledge.

He was a great big laughing man, always in good form, vital and vigorous, and his patients would say they felt better just looking at him; coming in to see him, they weren't just coming to see any doctor, but someone who knew their seed, breed and generation. The comfort of being listened to and understood, the warmth of a smile, these things can't be seen or touched or counted or measured, but they are very, very real. A lot of important things are like that.

I reflected on my good fortune; too many of our older generation are allowed to dream away their valuable experience while nodding by the fireside.

I'd never had a mentor, perhaps because I was too obnoxious; but also, I never thought I needed one, and it was an epiphany, after all the years of medical school and hospital and GP rotations, to encounter someone I could really admire and really want to emulate.

Without his guidance and example, I would have missed many things; how good it is to be needed, that it was better to like my patients than have them liking me, and most of all, the importance of being kind.

In his eighties, made weak by time and fate, we took a day-trip to Cheltenham National Hunt Festival. We left at the crack of dawn, took an early flight, had a wonderful day, walking the course beforehand, meeting the legends of the turf, relishing the gladiatorial atmosphere.

Exhausted, I dropped him back to his front door just before midnight, and then he turned to me, as if to strive, to seek, and not to yield, and said: 'That was great, young fella. Next year we'll go for the whole three days.'

Dedicated to the memory of Dr Jack Crummie

Making abortion legal, accessible and safe

GP 25 April 2018

In 1966, Romania, under Nicolai Ceausescu, decided that the Romanian population should be increased from 23m to 30m inhabitants. Decree 770 was authorised, and abortion and contraception declared illegal. To enforce the decree, contraceptives disappeared from the shelves, any detected pregnancies were closely followed until birth, and the secret police-maintained surveillance on procedures in hospitals.

This might sound draconian, but we don't have to look too far for parallels. The 1967 UK Abortion Act was never extended to Northern Ireland, and abortion remains illegal here.

We also have harsh criminal penalties; in theory life imprisonment for any woman undergoing an unlawful abortion. It's not just theory; a mother who helped her 15-year-old daughter procure abortion pills online is awaiting trial, and a number of women have faced prosecution within the last few years.

And when it comes to repudiating women's rights, we already have a virtual United Ireland. In the Republic of Ireland, the 8th Amendment to the constitution was introduced in 1983, giving equal weight to the life of the mother and that of the foetus. This has resulted in travesties such as the X Case; in 1992 a High Court ruling prevented a 14-year-old rape victim from travelling to England for an abortion.

These restrictive laws don't prevent abortions, as every year thousands of Irish women, north and south, make the lonely journey across the Irish Sea, and thousands of others order abortion pill online + take them without any medical supervision. According to a report by the Guttmacher Institute abortion rates are similar in countries where abortion is highly restricted and where it is broadly legal.

A more humane and effective approach for real 'pro-life' advocates would be to reduce the incidence of abortion by:

- improving sex education and access to contraception

- supporting women during pregnancy and child-rearing

- supporting disabled children and their families. In all my years as a family doctor, I don't ever recall any 'pro-life' advocates helping out in their care and giving exhausted and desperate parents a break.

Restrictions do have the effect of making abortion not only more expensive and distressing, but also more unsafe and less likely to be medically supervised, eroding trust between doctors and patients. Can a woman in crisis approach her doctor for help? Doctors are also placed in an invidious position. How can I ensure my patient is referred to a reputable clinic? How can I provide aftercare? How can I record it in my patient's file? How can I assure the woman that she is not facing this crisis alone?

But in at least one part of the island the times may be changing. On May 25th there will a referendum on repeal of the 8th Amendment, and perhaps at last recognition that you cannot legislate to compel a woman to carry a pregnancy to term, and that abortion must be legal, accessible, safe and free.

At this stage it looks as if the repeal motion is most likely to pass, but after the disasters of Brexit and Trump, there is no room for complacency. A woman must have the right to choose and to have control over her own body.

Footnote; This column is dedicated to Grace, my fervently pro-repeal daughter. Campaigning with her was an unexpectedly emotional experience, watching her passion and her determination to engage with every passerby, to secure every single vote.

Footnote 2; The referendum was passed by an overwhelming majority, 66% vs 33%.

The time of the buffoon has come

GP 12 July 2016

Joe is a member of the Dunning-Kruger club. The Dunning-Kruger effect is a cognitive bias in which relatively unskilled persons suffer illusory superiority, mistakenly assessing their ability to be much higher than it really is, and unable to recognize their own ineptitude and evaluate their own ability accurately; i.e you're so stupid you don't know how stupid you are.

'I need antibiotics, I've an awful sore throat,' said Joe. A regular request, but delivered in what I noticed was an unusually triumphalist tone.

Because I am sometimes A Good Doctor, I examined Joe's throat yet again (I could find my way around it in the dark). As usual it was clean as water imported from the rainforest with dolphins in it.

'It's probably a virus…' I began.

'I need antibiotics,' he insisted.

'Expert advice suggest that antibiotics are unnecessary in these cases,' I said.

'The British people are tired of listening to experts,' said Joe.

'So you're British now,' I said. 'But last month when Ireland beat Italy you were running down the street with the green flag wrapped around you.'

'Irish, British, whatever,' he said airily. 'I want my country back.'

'More specifically, I want my border back,' and then, in a far-away voice, full of yearning and nostalgia for times that will never come again: 'Smuggling diesel, cigarettes, videos, my old Transit van was like a brother to me; those were the days, my friend.

'There was a time,' I said sadly, 'when we aspired to intelligence, we weren't afraid of it.'

'You're yesterday's man, doc,' he said. 'Get with the zeitgeist. This is the era of Boris, of The Donald; the time of

75

buffoon politics has come. Buffoons get the press coverage, the name recognition, reality and surreality become blurred. Rational debate becomes impossible, because debating with nonsense only lends it credibility, so even the most outrageous claims go unchallenged. £350m ploughed into the NHS every week, stick it on the side of a bus; what kind idiot would fall for that?'

The first rule of the Dunning-Kruger club is that you don't know you're a member of the Dunning-Kruger club.

Aliens are people

GP 8 November 2017

'I'm an alien,' he said.

'That doesn't matter to me,' I said. 'That you are an immigrant, a refugee, and alien, whatever, is irrelevant; you are a human, I am a doctor. We treat everyone, that is our vocation, and in a world of avarice and fear and Trump and Brexit and suspicion of the outsider, it remains a noble vocation.'

'Not that kind of alien,' he explained, pushing a little button on his watch; his image shimmered for a moment, then two antennae sprouted from his head.

'We have to use a disguise,' he said, waggling his antennae. 'Don't want scare the native population; you know, anal probes and all.'

'I'm a bit vague on alien physiology,' I admitted.

'I knew it,' he said. 'I wanted to see a specialist but apparently I have to see a family doctor first; what would a family doctor know about aliens?'

'Very little,' I agreed. 'And as specialties fracture into subspecialties we know less and less about more and more; very soon we'll know nothing about everything.'

'Why do I need a referral anyway?' he protested. 'On my planet, if we get sick and have to take a break from the anal probing for a while, we can go directly to a specialist. If I have a cough, I go to a respirologist, if I have a hernia I go to a general surgeon (that's pretty much all they can do nowadays).'

This was a really good question, which forced me to confront the bleak reality of general practice.

'Because,' I explained, 'if everyone could just go and see a specialist whenever they wanted, the specialist would be seeing too many people with nothing wrong with them, and soon wouldn't be specialists at all. Orthopaedic surgeons would be overwhelmed by back pains, urologists by bladder infections, neurologists by headaches. They'd be seeing too much shite; it's our job to protect them from the shite; we see the shite and sift it out so the specialists don't have to see the shite. Some have romanticised our role; the Thin Red Line, The Watchers at the Gate, a pudgy, middle class Horatius at the bridge. But really we are just there to stop the shite; we are the Great Constipators of Healthcare.'

'Yeah, yeah,' he said. 'I've an awful sore throat, can you give me a prescription?'

Some truths are not just universal but inter-galactic, I reflected.

Another fine mess

BMJ 3 April 1999

'Who would have thought the old man to have had so much blood in him,' said Lady Macbeth; we sense her unrelenting ambition beginning to ebb and I reckon that Shakespeare must have been painfully conversant with both the spiritual and practical import of spilt blood. It can be a cathartic sight, and it makes a spectacle totally disproportionate to the amount bled.

Just the smallest drop can masquerade as a life-threatening haemorrhage. 'Don't be such a big baby, it's only a wee scratch,' we say, coincidently both withering and re-assuring, but even as we speak the mess on the floor, palpably sufficient to turn the multitudinous seas incarnadine, is making a barefaced liar out of us.

I was a casualty officer in the early 80s and in those days unless you were steeped in gore up to the armpits, you weren't cool. Blood held no atavistic terrors for us doctors, if somebody vomited blood over you it was a lot less revolting than somebody vomiting vomit. AIDS was as yet unknown, the first reports of GRIDs (Gay Related Immunity Disorders) were just coming though from the west coast of the United States, the rumble of distant thunder at a picnic.

The bogey then was hepatitis B, especially after the junior doctors in a Colin Douglas novel started dying like Greek flies who have indulged in multiple sexual indiscretions with blood relatives in a play by Aristophanes. Even so, we wore gloves even less often than condoms, and would ridicule the lab technicians who, if they pricked themselves, would need months of sick leave, counselling, cuddling, cosseting, and ultimately compensation.

In contrast, we were real men, we were immortal, invulnerable, too important and too vital to get sick, or so our dysfunctional culture told us.

The last time I shed blood myself, however involuntarily, I was almost proud. It was rich and crimson and sumptuous, a stark defiant shout of virility, a reaffirmation of the sheer indomitability and exuberance of life, the Red of Red Riding Hood, the biological equivalent of a Pepsi Cola advertisement.

'Lo, see what a miracle I am,' it trumpeted, 'I live, I breathe, I bleed.'

It is, after all, the second most romantic body fluid.

Vomiting... a joy forever

BMJ 8 May 1999

Andrew Lloyd Webber musicals, drugs reps personally demonstrating thixotropic nasal sprays; the world is full of unattractive things, and vomiting is reckoned among the worst of them.

Vomiting and the presence of a vomiting centre in the brain seems like yet more arguments against the existence of a benevolent God. There are other physical activities with better public relations which perhaps seem more deserving of a centre of their own, and in Thomas More's *Utopia*, all other methods of elimination were recognised as being among the pleasures of the flesh; he seems to have specifically excluded vomiting, perhaps to further annoy Henry VIII.

I can understand this attitude, however misguided it is, as I myself have vomited once or twice, and it wasn't pleasant. But to a physiologist, vomiting is actually an exquisitely elegant and fascinating manoeuvre, and there are irrefutably positive aspects to driving the porcelain bus.

Vomiting is divided into three parts; first of all nausea, you feel you want to vomit; then comes retching, all the sound effects and tumult and all the unique sensations— but nothing comes out; sound and fury, signifying nothing. Finally, the real thing… the vomit. The stomach starts to dance, the valves open, and whoop, up it comes, a wild trumpet blast on the unfortunate palate, and you think, 'I don't remember eating that.'

But no pain without gain, and vomiting is in fact a protective mechanism to get rid of poisons in a determinedly unforgettable manner; you might forget your birthday or anniversary, even your last columbine kiss, but nobody forgets their last vomit, or the circumstances which caused it. Such a complex activity requires part of the brain all to itself; the vomiting centre is devoted to coordinating the messages coming in from the stomach and the blood, and to sending them back to the stomach telling it to throw up immediately and damn the embarrassment. It's coincidently a great way of getting rid of unwanted company.

So the next time you get on the great white telephone to God, transcend the misery and remember that your body is presenting you with a most precious gift; emerald and ruby, amethyst and amber, a liquid bird of paradise, a spectacular, technicolour yawn, only Cecil B DeMille could direct the movie. A thing of beauty is…

Footnote; 'Thixotropic' means that the stuff sticks to the inner lining of the nose, not nice.

Health vs healthcare, and precision medicine

GP 3 October 2017

The first rule of Health Club is don't talk about health. Any discussion on health quickly morphs into a discussion on healthcare, though the two are quite different things. Healthcare only contributes to approximately 10% of health, 90% being due to the social determinants, education, sanitation, housing and above all poverty (I read that somewhere, so it must be true); Richard Smith observed that the main contribution of the NHS to population health was in providing employment.

And healthcare is trying to square the circle of ever-expanding needs, unrealistic expectations and limited resources. Every advance in medical science only augments the burden and makes the task even more unachievable; the more successful healthcare is, the more impossible it becomes. To paraphrase Somerset Maughan: 'There are three rules for designing a healthcare system. Unfortunately, no one knows what they are.'

And as resources are sucked into healthcare, everything else suffers, the environment, stand-up comedy, sports, everyone having a dog and learning the banjo, the arts, our schools, those things which do much more to enrich and lengthen life and reduce suffering than medicine and doctors and hospitals.

Healthcare can't be approached like an all-you-can-eat buffet, everyone grabbing whatever they can as quickly as possible whether they need it or not. Hard choices have to be made, but the right choices are always the hard ones (otherwise, everyone would always do the right thing).

Instead of, for example, ensuring that proven treatments are provided to everyone that needs them, there is always something new out of Africa...

'I'd like some precision medicine,' said Joe.

'Indeed,' I said.

'From now on,' he continued, 'I'd like my treatment to take into account the individuality of my genes, environment, and lifestyle. I'm tired of the one-size-fits-all approach, in which disease treatment and prevention strategies are developed for the average person, with less consideration for the differences between individuals. I am not Mr Average, I am unique, a child of the Universe, my very atoms forged in a dying star, noble in reason, infinite in faculties, in form and moving like an angel, in apprehension like a god.'

'No problem, Joe, here it is,' I said. 'There's precisely nothing wrong with you.'

Bad smells are good

BMJ 2 March 2002

I'm pretty hardy, and not overly sensitive to bad smells; delicacy is not a virtue in this job. Humans can apparently distinguish up to 10,000 different scents, which is useful for docs, as each body fluid has its own distinct aroma, and when these have been percolating for a few weeks or more they can become a heady brew.

Smegma, the stuff from infected sebaceous cysts, really stale urine, navel fluff that has been there for a generation, dead bodies, steatorrhoea, purulent phlegm, bad teeth—eight or nine pungent patients during an afternoon surgery on a warm day and the room becomes quite unforgettable.

Not all strong smells are unpleasant. Horse manure (or is it cow dung—can anyone tell the difference?) can be quite invigorating, a good honest reek, like going for a tramp across the fields, a whisper of the countryside to sweeten even the darkest and most drear surgery.

Smells should indeed be our friends; open your arms and welcome them in. They are such a valuable form of non-verbal communication—for example, 'You are only the doctor and not worth getting cleaned up for.' They are also an intrinsic part of the diagnostic process, as with the patient who smelled as if he had been marinated overnight in cat's widdle.

'Do you have a cat?' I asked shrewdly, sending off the toxoplasma titre.

'How did you know?' he gasped.

'Just a wild guess,' I said, nodding sagely, like Sherlock Holmes' patronising well-meaning but bumbly Dr Watson.

Watson was no role model for me, I preferred Doc Holliday, lean, hungry, doomed, dangerous, decadent, and cynical though he was; he had that touch of fatal glamour, and I bet he smelled of whisky, cigars, and cologne.

Smell is more tenacious than the other senses; get it on your skin and even if you scrub and scrub and scrub you are not washing it off, merely spreading it around, like Lady Macbeth's dread spot. It is more resistant to time. When the Catman left the room, though his corporeal body was gone, his presence yet hovered around me like a forlorn and stinky little ghost; the song was over, but the memory lingered on, a gift to soften my regret at our parting, also to be savoured by other patients, who probably thought that I was the one with the cat problem.

And if some of them did happen to gag, it certainly made them forget the complaint they came in with, which is practically the same thing as a cure, isn't it?

GUBU: grotesque, unbelievable, bizarre, unprecedented

BMJ 18 November 2004

'I don't really know what to say, doc,' said Joe.

I closed my eyes in resignation; could he be any more ambiguous?

One of the skills in general practice is defining the problem. Anything, just anything, can walk though that surgery door. Tragic, comic, or unremittingly trivial—it's our job to reduce it to some form of manageable problem. But in terms of vagueness and sheer unhelpfulness it's hard to beat that opening gambit.

Country practice, though, has its advantages, and I already had an important clue. That same network of family, friends, and neighbours that lends such support in times of crisis has a dark side: in the Valley of the Squinting Windows nothing is missed, and at a recent football match Joe had been reported as walking funny.

A few questions further defined the problem. We men are simple creatures; we hate to lose face, and Joe claimed to have haemorrhoids the shape and size of the Mountains of the Moon—not usually the kind of thing one boasts about, even to one's best mates.

A rectal exam was indicated, but as I palpated, I felt a GUBU coming on—a big, big sneeze. What with my hands being both occupied and repulsive, there was no way to hold my nose or grab a hanky. I tried wrinkling my nose, tried supratentorial over-ride (it works for hiccups, as also, curiously, does digital rectal massage); I begged the gods for succour, but the gods are capricious and hate doctors because people trust us and we are a big hit with the girls.

'Wazoo,' I screamed, catarrh exploding across the room. The elemental force of the blast was stunning, almost like an orgasm but without the emotional commitment, and left me in awe of my body's musculature: such power, such elegance, such coordination.

It is the small details I still remember of that climactic moment: the beat of opalescent body fluids on pearly white Irish buttocks that haven't seen much sunshine and have therefore remained commendably youthful and free of wrinkles, Joe's squeal of protest as an already uncomfortable experience became suddenly a disturbing one, the attending nurse's auburn hair wafting in the gale, reminding me of those Woody Allen comedies about autumn in New York.

'I don't really know what to say,' I said.

'Sure hope that was just a sneeze, doc,' said Joe.

Let's get naked

GP 18 April 2012

Farrell's 2nd Law; the longer it takes for a patient to disrobe, the less likely there is to be any significant clinical finding.

There is obviously a huge cost implication for the NHS here. Instead of sitting there twiddling our thumbs or daydreaming or idly googling to see what Britney Spears is up to, while Mrs Murphy laboriously removes corset number four with a hammer and chisel, we could be doing something useful.

But I have a solution; some might consider it rather extreme, but at a stroke it would rectify this drain on scarce resources; we should all get naked.

OK, OK, I hear you say, some of it won't be pretty, have we not suffered enough?

But think of all the time we'd save. Because it wouldn't just be patients; to maintain a balance in the doctor-patient relationship, doctors would have to get naked as well.

No need to worry any more about what suit to wear, whether our trousers are pressed, which tie goes with which shirt - a major source of stress would be history.

There would also be less tangible, more spiritual rewards. Clothes have lost their traditional purpose - to keep us warm and dry - instead, our culture has become so trivial that clothes have become a statement, a status symbol.

Getting naked would liberate us from these pretensions, get us closer to the truth of who we really are; here I am, we'd say, this is me, I am a child of the universe, peace, love and rock'n'roll, this is my glorious naked body, no longer fettered by fashion and convention, and of which I am not ashamed.

The rest of society would also benefit. Going through security at airports would be a breeze; no more being herded into long queues like sheep, no more having to take off shoes and coats and belts, we'd be straight in there to the duty free and the free samples of expensive aftershave.

Terrorists would have nowhere to hide their paraphernalia; well, maybe there's one place, so a lot more rectals would be needed, but they're not that bad, and can even be quite pleasant.

If performed by an attractive person, that is.

The flagon... with the dragon

BMJ 13 October 2005

It was more than just a heart-sink consultation; it was tedious, nagging, grating, the kind of consultation that whispers the o'erwrought heart and bids it break. 'You are in perfect health, Mrs Maguire,' I repeated.

'Are you sure I'm all right?'

'I'm sure.'

'Are you definitely sure?'

'Definitely.'

'Are you absolutely definitely sure?'

'Absolutely.'

'Are you absolutely definitely positively sure?'

'When was the last time someone actually hit you?' Of course I didn't say that; I was too busy gouging a scalpel into my left inner thigh and lapsing into my old defence mechanism of mumbling classic comedy sketches. 'The pellet with the poison's in the vessel with the pestle, the chalice from the palace has...'

'I beg your pardon,' she said.

'I'm sorry,' I said, 'Did I say that out loud?'

'In any case,' she said, 'there's been a change; the chalice is broken, they've had to replace it with a flagon.'

'With a flagon?' I said, surprised.

'With the figure of a dragon.'

'The flagon with the dragon,' I mused.

'Yes,' she said, 'The vessel with the pestle has the pellet with the poison, the flagon with the dragon…'

'… has the brew that is true,' we shouted in unison, laughing and jumping up and down with excitement.

It was like being on the Road to Damascus while riding a bike for the first time and losing your virginity, all in one glorious blast; patient is too small a word, patients aren't one dimensional, I realised, they are real people with families, friends, lovers, jobs, passions. And Mrs Maguire's passion, I found out, was Hollywood comedies, pre-1960.

'Your proposition may be good…' I ventured, in an homage to Groucho,

'…but let's have one thing understood.' She was right with me, then, altogether, 'Whatever it is, I'm against it.'

We spent an agreeable last few minutes sparring over the relative merits of *Bringing Up Baby* and *The Man Who Came to Dinner*.

'By the way,' she said, 'I've an awful sore throat; can I have an antibiotic?'

I looked at her, a trifle disappointed; had our time together meant nothing?

'Just yanking your chain doc,' she said, deadpan.

Footnote; This is my favourite piece; my love of old movies and one of the secrets being a good doctor.

The unbearable inadequacy of language

BMJ 21 December 1996

James Thurber once lamented the existence of those things, actions, expressions, situations, etc, which exist but have not yet been named—for example, to try and avoid someone in the street by stepping to one side. Your adversary mirrors your movements and together you shuffle from side to side in a bizarre little dance, both desperately trying to get past the other. Eventually you extricate yourselves with an embarrassed smile and go on your way. Recognise the situation? There's no word for it.

Medicine is particularly affected by this insufficiency of nomenclature, so we at the BMJ have decided to take urgent corrective action, and today we make a few suggestions of how these lost meanings could be usefully married to Irish place names, which otherwise do nothing but loaf around on signposts scratching themselves.

Moy (noun): a small papilloma which the owner regularly plays with. 'Worried by the news of his mother in law's hernia, Maguire absently played with his moy.'

Limavady (n): the irresistible desire to incise an abscess. 'The cyst was swollen and pointing and he felt a limavady coming on.'

Leitrim (n): an E. Coli UTI which is sensitive to trimethoprim. By common usage this term has expanded to refer to all extremely rare medical events—for example, an objective medicolegal report, a dentist who is actually available for emergencies.

Nenagh (n): an unconsummated limavady—that is, when no pus comes shooting out, no matter how much you hack and hack and hack. A disappointing feeling.

Belfast (n): a patient who appears at the surgery door even before your finger has touched the buzzer. 'Only 11am on Monday morning, and he'd already had three belfasts.'

Lislea (verb): the skill by which complimentary biros disappear so quickly. One theory is that they slip through a worm hole in space and end up on the planet Bartowel, where they have developed a sophisticated civilisation, and may soon invade earth. Consequently, the theory runs, all biros should be treated with kindness (remember the whales in Star Trek IV?).

Killough (v): to cough vigorously outside the surgery door, to let the doctor know you are waiting, that you are impatient, and that you are really sick. Often employed by a belfast (qv).

Comber (v): to copy all the references from a review article and pretend you've actually looked them up yourself.

Burren (n): some other poor bugger's work.

Ennis (v): (patient) to remove one's sock with a snapping motion, thereby expelling a shower of stale sweat and flakes of dead skin into the doctors' face. "Beware of the ennis,' Professor Gregorivich told his awed students, 'And always have a towel handy." Anton Chekhov, Uncle Vanya

Derry (v): to present a burren (qv) with deceitful sincerity. Professors and heads of department are good at this. 'At the meeting in Monte Carlo burren after burren was derried by a panel of distinguished speakers.'

Cullybackey (n): a scientific paper in which there are more authors than subjects. The New England Journal specialises in these. 'This week five interesting cully-backies throw a new light on gerbils as disease vectors.' New England Journal of Medicine.

Cooley (v): to add one's name to a research paper, despite having done none of the work. Part of the process which facilitates a derry (qv) and results ultimately in a cully-backy (qv). To cooley has recently become rather disreputable but what the hell, who's going to know.

Hoddity (n): trite indulgent poetry in a medical journal, particularly *The Lancet*. 'A hoddity is like a dog shaking hands; it is not done well, but one is surprised to see it done at all.' Dr Samuel Johnson.

Footnote; Douglas Adams, writer of *The Hitch-hikers Guide to the Galaxy,* had recently published *The Meaning of Liff* which gave me the idea for this article. I wrote to him and asked permission to use this literary device and received a dismissive letter from his agent. But when I looked into it further, Lewis Carroll and James Thurber had used it before him, so what the heck.

Footnote 2; In honour of the deceased author, a new 20th anniversary edition of *The Meaning of Liff* was published; I submitted an entry and received a free copy in payment. Nice......

Smug

BMJ 27 February 1999

'OK, OK, send her in and we'll take a look at her,' said the junior hospital doctor, his tone pregnant with studied insolence.

'Don't patronise me, you smug little shit,' I felt like saying, 'I was looking after sick kids before you were masturbating.'

But I didn't, because I was that soldier, and neither would you, because we've all been there, haven't we; brainwashed, either overtly or insidiously, all through medical school, that GPs are lazy and stupid.

At his age he won't understand. He is young, and to him so much is occult and mysterious. Why are we here? What was Woodstock and was there really a band called Country Joe and the Fish? What do health visitors do? What is the meaning of life? Why do small bald men always want to become surgeons? Can Darth Vader really be Luke Skywalker's father?

But if I could I would kiss his lips and take his hand and sit him down among long dappled grass and explain the recherché perversity of general practice; how it is not a specialty, but rather a generality, with all the burdens and privileges that this role confers, demanding skills that reach across the divide, not just of a dissonant phalanx of fragmented medical specialties, but of that deep romantic chasm between science and art, haunted by woman wailing for her demon lover.

If we truly have any special interest or skill it is in understanding the individual, surely the most Daedaelian subject of all. As Voltaire said, 'It is easier to understand Mankind than to understand one man.'

We are the Corinthians, the Renaissance Men, the profession of Chekhov and Turgenev, empathic students and observers of the human condition, so close your eyes in holy dread, lad, for we on honeydew have fed and drunk the drink of paradise.

The call of the wild (rabbit)

BMJ 10 June 1995

The BMJ Christmas issue reported cases of squirrel and mouse bites but I can do much better than that.

A patient came in recently with a rabbit bite, I kid you not. If the abrasion had been any more superficial it would have been protuberance. Laying on the antiseptic as thick as the sarcasm, I admonished him sternly.

'Were you teasing it with a stick?' I asked, 'or putting your hand in and out of its mouth to impress your friends?'

Our prehistoric ancestors survived by hunting down small furry creatures, and attractive though this sounds, rabbit meat is no longer an essential part of our diet. But not wanting to be too flippant, and just in case I had missed something, I requested a Medline search on rabbit-induced trauma.

My search was fruitless; apparently, even in a pack, even if reared by wolves, and even if cornered, rabbits will not attack humans. Like Stout Cortez, I could wildly surmise only a danger that might come from the rabbits' admirably vegetarian diet; some minerals, vitamins, and fibre might have inadvertently leached into the abrasion, there causing an unprecedented surge of rude health which the patient's sedentary lifestyle and cafeteria diet would be unable to sustain.

On the same day I received a call to a young man with a productive cough; on arrival I found him sitting on the edge of the bed, video and TV remote controls immediately to hand, and looking inappropriately healthy.

When I asked what colour his phlegm was he pointed to a revolting smudge on the floor.

'You can see for yourself, doc,' he said; here's one I prepared earlier' (OK, I made that last sentence up) as he once again hawked enthusiastically, reminding me perversely of Browning's wise thrush;

'Who sings each song twice over/Lest you think he never could recapture/That first fine careless rapture.'

The moment

BMJ 9 August 1997

Last year, while skiing, my friends and I fell into the company of some German folk. They seemed pleased at first, their reserve perhaps balanced by our more extrovert nature. Gradually, however, you could sense their perspective changing, and the realisation dawning that they had not encountered a tableau of richly Joycean characters but rather a bunch of obnoxiously drunken buffoons.

There is a thin line between love and hate, but an even shorter step from entertainer to pest; the hero can become the zero in the blink of an eye.

El Gran Senor was thought to be a champion; but in that seminal moment two furlongs out, Pat Eddery went for his whip and found—nothing. The garrulous patient that keeps you entertained for ten minutes till you realise he is a manic depressive; the patient who attends many times with non-specific general complaints till the penny drops in a chilling instant that there is probably a malignancy present.

Unfortunately, this moment of enlightenment is often imperceptible.

The pivotal nature of continuing care by a single doctor is one of the more sensible mantras of academic general practice. When I was an intern the team consisted of a consultant, a senior registrar, a research registrar, a senior house officer on rotation, a senior house officer not on rotation (a particularly pathetic species), two other interns, and about 60 cajillion medical students, and still nobody knew anything about the patients.

But there is a Dark Side; familiarity can obscure any gradual changes and prevent us from recognising these critical moments. Our concept of time is too coarse; when we look in the mirror each day we don't see ourselves growing older, and similarly, if we see a patient too often all but the most obvious changes are invisible.

Then that infuriating, inevitable day comes when the partner/locum/consultant, blessed with the fresh, unprejudiced eye, says: 'Hey, that guy's a classic case; how did you miss that he is hypothyroid/acromegalic/growing two heads?'

Well, it's easy to miss it, you smug bastards, and your time will come. The second head starts as a tiny bump, classically on the right shoulder where the parrot usually sits; two weeks later it's a wee bit bigger, then slowly over the years it grows until before you know it, like Robert Browning envying you guys waking in England and seeing one morning, 'unaware/That the lowest boughs of the brushwood sheaf/Round the elm-tree bole are in tiny leaf,' you've got a fully grown second head giving you cheeky backtalk.

By now a simple, painless cure is no longer possible. The axe must be scalpel sharp, or else you will have to hack and hack and hack and hack, just like when you butcher a hog, and all the while the second head is ducking and weaving, alternatively screaming and cursing and cajoling and wheedling and trying to persuade you that you are cutting off the wrong head.

95

So if a frequent attender is having problems an early second opinion can be a smart move.

In medicine, two heads are definitely better than one.

I saw Satan fall like lightning

BMJ 8 April 2000

I was called recently to a patient who had collapsed in church. At church is a good place to collapse, implying a previous life of probity and devotion, and the bystanders are likely to be helpful. Collapsing outside a bar late at night, by contrast, you are unlikely to get a lift home from a friendly drug dealer; a better class of people attend church, although they may be more fastidious about mouth to mouth—perhaps not a bad thing. The doctor also feels more obliged to attend; there is something deserving about a church carpark. This collapse, we infer, is unrelated to debauchery.

I drove out at once, but some do-gooder had already taken the patient to the surgery. And, returning to the surgery, I found, with a certain fatal satisfaction, that the entourage had inevitably returned to the church.

Eventually, a few laps later, I hounded the patient to earth. Invigorated by the chase, she was at first unwilling to accept cardiac pulmonary resuscitation, but a crowd had gathered and, as Pierre said in *War and Peace*, the common good is the only kind there is. Pleasing the mob always comes first, and saying all was fine would have been inconsiderately detumescent; doing nothing was too hard a proposition, the power was intoxicating, put a beggar on horseback and he'll ride to hell.

So, instead a symphony; excited oohs as I whip out the shock blanket like a magician's rabbit; somebody shouting, 'Don't move her!' (mandatory); the triumphant clash of the defib paddles as I flourish them on high; the patient's futile protests, 'I'm fine, no really I am, really'; the crowd moaning and crooning and swaying with pleasure until the ambulance arrives, rabbits transfixed by the weasel's dance.

I accepted the plaudits modestly, and as I led her up the steps into the ambulance, its interior lambent like a little piece of heaven, a ghostly Roman slave appeared at my elbow, whispering, 'Memento mei tu es.'

Doctor/patient relationship hits new low

GP 11 April 2014

Progress can be painful, but sacrifices must be made in the name of science. I took a deep breath, girded my loins and started morning surgery. I had diligently researched the correct technique and when Joe came in, I turned my back, reversed, adopted a squat and began wiggling my hips, while sticking my tongue out laterally as far as possible.

Greeting patients used to be simple. 'Hi', 'hello', a surly grunt, a nod of the head, or even, if you were feeling especially committed to Being A Good Doctor: 'How are you?'

Then these casual greetings were deemed patronising and a formal handshake became the required method; stuffy and time-consuming, although it could always be enlivened by smearing lubricating jelly on your hand first.

But academia moved on, looking for another grant, and hygiene became the imperative. Where had the patient's hand been, we had to wonder, which can be difficult to establish.

A whole hand-washing industry sprouted - international conferences, campaigns, advocates, inspectors, professors, lecturers, *et al.* Handshakes, the tide of history told us, were no longer advisable due to risk of spreading infection.

So let's take the hands out of the equation, I thought, and watching Miley Cyrus gave me the inspiration for a revolutionary and impeccably hygienic form of greeting: twerking.

While involving no skin-to-skin contact, it is the perfect introduction, creating the ambience for what will surely be a deeply intimate doctor/patient relationship. Like every scientific innovation, it will take a while for patients to get with the programme.

'Gotta say it, doc,' said Joe, 'that's pretty weird.'

'The worst is yet to come, Joe,' I replied. 'You have to do it to me now.'

Chapter 5

I'll just have an antibiotic, then

Some day you and I, and all the people we know, all the people we love, will die and slowly be forgotten. Dust we were, and dust we will return to, as civilizations rise and fall, oceans run dry and mountains crumble.

But some things never change, and the eternal struggle will go on; the desire of patients to take antibiotics, the heroic yet futile attempts of doctors to avoid prescribing them.

A tale of two Irish Mammies

GP 18 July 2016

In a referendum in Ireland last year, amid much rejoicing, same-sex marriage was approved, and Ireland moved another step away from its post-colonial Victorian prudery; we were previously a bawdy folk.

But as usual, there were unforeseen consequences, especially for doctors; one Irish Mammy is formidable enough, but some lucky boys and girls now have two Irish Mammies.

Irish Mammy(1) has for years waged an unrelenting and deeply personal war against childhood fevers. She knows every trick in the book, every strategy, and every route of attack (oral, axillary, and rectal), and as usual she began with a breathless hour by hour account of the previous night's skirmish

'Little Johnny's temperature was up at eight o'clock,' said Irish Mammy(1).

'We got it down by giving him Calpol, then it came up again, so at 22 hundred hours we ducked him in a bath of crushed ice and dead otters,' said Irish Mammy(2).

'Still it wouldn't come down, so we force-fed him some cold pureed hyena,' said Irish Mammy(1).

Little Johnny looked full of beans and had managed to get his head stuck in the sharps box, the Venus Fly-Trap bright colours of which were probably designed specially to attract young children to their doom. He was screaming, but this was, I reckoned, an appropriate response to his situation and a sign of general wellbeing.

'I have here,' I said, 'the very latest research from the National Institute for Health and Clinical Excellence. They are clever chaps, and their guidelines clearly state that fever is not necessarily a bad thing; indeed, experts say it may even help children fight infections.'

'The British people are tired...' began Irish Mammy(1).

'I know, I know,' I said, '...of listening to experts.'

The two Irish Mammies looked at each other, brows darkening at my heresy; I could see in their eyes a fanatical gleam, shadows of a burning stake and a lynch mob, and I noticed Irish Mammy(2) was wearing a sweatshirt with a tasteful swastika logo.

We doctors must step deftly along tangled paths, but I made my decision, I made my stand. Galileo and the Vatican, Salman Rushdie and the Ayatollah - I was just another small soldier in the eternal struggle against intolerance and bigotry and unreason. Unknown, perhaps, and unrenowned, but no less valorous and worthy of honour.

'They further state,' I continued steadfastly, 'that antipyretic treatments, such as paracetamol and ibuprofen, are not recommended.'

Irish Mammy(1) gave a little gasp, her temples crashing down in ruin all around her.

'Also,' I said, aware that I was challenging a whole belief system, 'physical measures, such as ice baths and tepid sponging, are not recommended.'

Irish Mammy(1) appeared quelled, but my victory was but a fleeting jade, as Irish Mammy(2) rose in triumph from the wreckage of her fallen idols.

'We'll just have an antibiotic then,' she said.

Smart-phone consultations; the bright side......

GP 21 November 2017

In medicine, as in life, even when nothing is happening, something is happening.

I hadn't seen Joe for a while; he had a carnival of complaints, all of which he'd have googled and catastrophised about beforehand, so you might consider the cessation of his daily visits as a most welcome development, like the relief you feel when you stop banging your head against a brick wall.

But as Hitchcock said: 'There is no terror in the bang, only in the anticipation of it.' I was getting anxious, waiting for the other shoe to drop, and for Joe to descend upon me in wrath with a Ragnarok of symptomatology.

So when I passed his cottage, quaintly decorated with the traditional Irish aluminium windows and Sky satellite dish, I thought I'd check him out.

He seemed a bit furtive.

'There is a kind of confession in your looks,' I said, 'which your modesties have not craft enough to colour.'

'OK, OK, I was dreading having to tell you,' said Joe. 'There's no easy way to say this, I know it'll hurt, but I'll be straight; I've got myself another doctor.'

Ignoring my little jig of despair, he pulled out his mobile phone.

'Look at this,' he said. 'Doc in My Pants, it's called. 'See an NHS GP in minutes', they said. Now I can talk to a doctor whenever I want. They're available any time of the day, any time of the night, 24/7.

'And so am I, my Precioussss,' he added, his tone both sinister and self-satisfied.

He pressed a button and a screen came up. 'Symptom checker,' it said.

'You're supposed to go through this first,' explained Joe. 'To see if you really need to see a doctor at all, but everyone just skips that part. Self-limiting disorders, I don't think so.'

A new screen appeared, a harassed young doc, who I noted was wearing a stethoscope, purely for theatrical purposes, I presume, but we all do that, don't we?

'Not you again,' he said to Joe, before getting up and walking off-screen. There was a banging sound which the experienced clinician could instantly recognise as the head of an exasperated colleague making repeated contact with a brick wall.

'You see,' said Joe. 'They already know me well.'

That's continuing care for you, I thought.

Cars: the bluffer's guide

GP 18 February 2010

We doctors suffer from something described as the 'extension of incompetence'. Because of our carefully hoarded knowledge about the human body and stuff, and the resultant status afforded us by society, we are also presumed to be wise in other areas, legal, financial, geological etc. And, of course, mechanical.

Last week, I came upon Joe broken down by the side of the road (his car was broken down, I mean).

As there was nothing good on TV and I felt that after a tough morning surgery, I deserved some free entertainment (did I mention it was raining heavily?), I stopped to have a closer look.

The usual crowd had gathered to offer unwanted advice, but when Joe saw my arrival, his face lit up.

'Doctor,' he said, 'what do you think?'

Now, I know as much about car engines as I do about interpreting electrolyte lab results, but I haven't got where I am today by being unable to cover up that I haven't got a clue what I'm talking about.

So I had a stock phrase ready and prepared for this very situation, partly inspired by the Father Ted episode where Fr Jack is conditioned to respond to every question with: 'That would be an ecumenical matter.'

I kicked the tyres (because some conventions must be observed), then leaned over the engine, scowled as if disgusted by what I was looking at, and then asked: 'Did you try the carburettor?'

A satisfied murmur went through the crowd and Joe said: 'I hadn't thought of that.'

Gratified by the reaction, I allowed myself an encore.

'Could be water in the carburettor,' I opined solemnly. The bucketing rain grew even heavier, adding gravity to my words, none of which, you will note, were directive, but had been couched in general terms, giving me an escape clause and absolving me of any responsibility for the outcome.

'Of course, I'd need to look underneath,' looking around yearningly as if my dearest wish was for a water-proof tarpaulin so I could crawl under the engine, while simultaneously triggering my phone to ring and pretending to answer it.

'Rats, an emergency, gotta go right now,' I said, squelching away quickly. 'My work here is done.'

The despair of differential diagnoses

GP 14 February 2014

'But soft! What light through yonder window breaks? It is the east, and Juliet is the sun.'

If a firm diagnosis was perched invitingly on that balcony, we family doctors wouldn't need ruby lips, a heaving bosom, a wanton come-hither gaze and golden hair hanging down to be equally as ardent. Once we have the diagnosis, management is a breeze, but all too often, we find the diagnosis fluttering far away from our despairing grasp.

With multiple conflicting, confusing symptoms raining down on me, rather than stick a fork in my eyeball out of sheer frustration, sometimes I try to zone out, stare at the spots on the wallpaper and try to count them, hoping that my subconscious will take a break from its obsession with sex and actually help out for once (there are 342 spots, by the way, 343 if you include the smudge caused by one of Joe's more spectacular expectorations).

Unfortunately, 'I haven't the faintest clue what's wrong with you, but it's probably nothing serious and will get better on its own, so be cool, baby,' doesn't count as a diagnosis. The Irish version, 'Feck it, sure it'll be grand,' is more elegant and succinct, and patients seem to find it reassuring; it's diagnosis and prognosis all in one, maybe it could be adopted more widely, perhaps even incorporated into the Liverpool Care Pathway.

Joe was a constant challenge. His symptoms were vague, never any coherent pattern, and would have left even dear old Mr Harrison and his two-ton *Principles of Internal Medicine* scratching his head.

Today was no different; a general 'uneasy' feeling that someone was following him, numbness here and there, and floaters which were apparently affecting his ability to enjoy online porn.

But I haven't been a GP for years without developing a certain low cunning. 'Have you ever had this before?' I asked.

'Yes,' he said helpfully, as precise as always, 'A few times, here and there, now and then.'

'Feck it,' I said, 'Sure it'll be grand.'

The scholar's tale

BMJ 30 June 2009

Many of the skills of general practice lie beyond the remit of mere medical science, though I am always circumspect about giving non-medical advice. 'Never criticise a brave until you have walked a mile in his moccasins,' goes the proverb, to which I might add: 'Especially if it's uphill on a hot day, the brave sweats a lot, he has a fungal foot infection and doubtful personal hygiene, and his moccasins are made out of recycled rubber tyres.'

But sometimes we have no choice. General practice is a broad church, because for some reason patients believe that our expertise extends into uncharted seas, where we must boldly go, and we never know what conundrum might next walk through that surgery door.

He was carrying a book, not unusual in itself, but the books are usually chick lit novels or thrillers or *Da Vinci Code* lookalikes (the shroud of Turin having been found by carbon dating to be a representation of St Paul cutting Lazarus's toenails, which had grown inconveniently long while he was dead, and the church's murderous attempts to keep this quiet lest the world should suddenly realise that all religion is basically mythological shite).

This was different: *The Divine Comedy*, no less, which was set down on my desk in an unspoken challenge. I consider myself well read (as a columnist I'm always looking out for someone to plagiarise), but this was intimidating.

The consultation seemed superficially normal: a sore throat, cough, and snuffles—the banality of evil, I reflected. But the dance was on; for a time we adeptly skirted the elephant in the room, but the final confrontation was inevitable.

'You are familiar with Dante?' he said at last, patronising as only a lay person can be. But under the pretext of calculating his cardiovascular risk (and we all know how useful and practical that is), I had done some emergency googling. Wikipedia, I have found, will never let you down; even if it's not always accurate, it's always plausible.

'Ah,' I said, 'We have reached the 10th circle of Hell.'

'I believe you are mistaken, doctor,' said the smartass, 'There were only nine circles.'

'Wrong, buddy,' I said, 'St Luke reserved the 10th circle for those who expect antibiotics for minor upper respiratory tract infections.'

'You got me there, doc,' he admitted.

'*Lasciate ogne speranza voi ch'intrate,*' I said.

Footnote; The final line is, of course, Dante's 'Abandon all hope, ye who enter here,' but you knew that already, I'm sure.

A Wheelbarrow of tablets.......

GP 2 August 2007

Each day in general practice is a battle, so I feel some empathy for the great warmongers. I look a map of Europe and wonder how Napoleon and Hitler didn't look at the same map and say 'F*ck me, look at the size of Russia, and they say the weather ain't good either; no way we're invading that place, let's check out Belgium again.'

A wise general chooses his battles carefully. Which is why I don't bother anymore trying to get old women off their tablets.

If Le Grande Armee couldn't do it and ended up getting cut to pieces by the Cossacks, what chance have I? But sometimes we can use this obstinacy to our advantage. Even the smallest victory should be celebrated.

Mrs Murphy was retching noisily and theatrically.

'I'm dying, I'm dying,' she wailed.

But I knew there was bugger-all wrong; there was no way a truly ill person could have come up with those incredible sound effects.

'Could I just check your tablets?' I said.

This is a useful technique; it gives us a few minutes breathing space, and the turn of phrase implies that we already know exactly what they are taking (knowledge which would require a brain the size of a planet) and that we want to ensure that compliance with their multi-drug regimen is correct.

A daughter-in-law wearily pushed in a small wheelbarrow, and I began to go through the bottles, a fascinating and multi-coloured cocktail of hypnotics, antidepressants, vitamins and analgesics, making small tut-tuts and disapproving grunts and occasionally murmuring: 'Mmm, very sickening, could be that one, or this one, maybe, it could choke a horse.'

The retching sounds behind me slowly abated as Mrs Magee began to realise my out-flanking stratagem.

'I'm feeling a little bit better now,' she said, just the right amount of tremor in her voice.

I shook the wheelbarrow in a vaguely threatening manner.

'Much better, in fact,' she said, rising from the bed like the morning sun and taking command of the wheelbarrow.

Conceding the battle, but, I admit, still winning the war.

Close encounters with an ingrowing toenail

GP 9 April 2018

I was holding the baby, or in this case, the toenail; over the years I had unwittingly earned the reputation of being good with toenails.

Joe's ingrowing toenail had a precious place on the crowded mantelpiece of our long and painful (painful for me, that is) relationship; unlovely though it was, it was the only objective evidence of a medical condition Joe had ever produced; everything else was just Joe's symptoms, i.e. lies.

Our diseases are not something distinct from us, they are part of what we are, and Joe's toenail was the cherry on top. I'd been hacking at it for years, and had even briefly considered decapitation, but the toenail and I had by now a personal relationship; perhaps we recognised each other as apex predators. As Ugarte said to Rick in Casablanca: 'Just because you despise me, you are the only one I trust.'

'Wotcha, mate,' the toenail seemed to say, 'Hear me roar,' as Joe snapped off his socks, showering me accidentally on purpose with a pungent bouquet of sweat and flakes of dead skin.

There's a reason the Body Shop doesn't have a line of products called Joe's Smelly Feet, but hey, I'm a doc, we're used to that stuff and bad smells and stale bodily fluids don't bother us.

Mostly.

After retching for a few short minutes, and cognisant of our special relationship, I set the toe on a little cushion; it was not quite Old Babylonian decadence, but at least a little less repulsive.

'Ah, look at the wee thing,' said Joe fondly. 'There sleeps Titania sometime of the night, Lull'd in these flowers with dances and delight.'

The toenail was minimally ingrowing; if had been any less ingrowing it would actually have been sticking out, but that was good enough for Joe; the minimal degree of ingrowingness allowed us to use our imaginations. As Patrick Kavanagh wrote: 'Through a chink too wide/There comes in no wonder.'

I gave it a respectful little massage and some antibiotics (what else?) and advised it to rest.

A minimal intervention perhaps, but I was content; we doctors, we do terrible things to toenails.

Do me a favour; no…

GP 30 May 2012

'Could you do me a favour?' asked Joe, leaning in close with a conspiratorial air, even more shifty than usual, which is saying a lot; Harry Lime could have taken lessons. I leaned back in reciprocal fashion, our little *pas de deux* a consequence of Joe's unique and compelling fragrance.

I'm not being abnormally fastidious in this regard, because no-one ever gets too close to Joe. Even at a crowded football match, Joe will stand aloof, a lonely little island.

I've never been involved in teaching undergraduates and my one lecture to GP trainees ended with me advising them to give up general practice and join the Foreign Legion because that way, they'd probably kill fewer people, so I haven't been asked back. But if given another chance, I would include a warning against the words 'Could you do me a favour?'

We are doctors; it goes without saying that we are trying to help our patients out. So being asked to do a favour always means that something extra is required, something outside the usual call of duty, some subterfuge which will involve a stretching of our moral fabric. And the more quietly it is asked, the more shady the plot, the more clandestine the manoeuvre, the more grave the misdemeanour that is demanded. The potential subjects are myriad; insurance, sick certs, DLA forms, planning applications, passport forms for potential underwear bombers etc etc, but there is one common theme; we are being asked to partake in a conspiracy, to corrupt the values of our ancient and noble profession.

But age has lent me wisdom, as well as haemorrhoids.

'A favour,' I said, returning the word like I was throwing back an unwanted fish.

'My neighbour's dog is barking all night and annoying me,' he said. 'And I thought maybe I could get a sick line, saying that it's making me depressed and all.'

Joe's neighbour, I knew, was a man with a reputation for extracting slow-burning yet inexorable vengeance. Taking a stance in the opposite camp would not be a smart move. For once, ethics and practicality were seamlessly wedded.

'I'm sorry, Joe,' I replied, the words rising unbidden, 'but you're barking up the wrong tree.'

Keeping things confidential

GP 25 January 2017

'Three men may keep a secret,' said Benjamin Franklin (while turning over in his grave at the election of Donald Trump), 'if two of them are dead.' Discretion can be tough, but patient confidentiality has always been a cornerstone of medical practice, and like every other family doctor, I hold many unwritten secrets which I will carry to my grave.

But when confidentiality is carried to extremes it becomes a paralysing force, making normal communication impossible. If the right hand doesn't know what the left hand is doing, how can they clap? There has to be a crack in everything, that's how the light gets in.

Joe was complaining of Symptom No 23(b), an 'awful' cough, a complaint which was as, usual, contradicted by his animal vigour and vitality, what the Trump administration would have called 'alternative facts', i.e lies.

'I'm worried about my confidentiality,' said Joe. 'When I'm in the waiting room, everyone else in the room knows I'm there as well. Not very confidential, is it? They're probably all talking about it.'

'Joe,' I said. 'Your arrival in the waiting room is like the sun coming up every morning, we have learned to rely upon it. In a time of chaos, fear and anti-intellectualism, in the era of Boris, Trump and Le Pen, it is comforting that some things never change.

'Indeed, your absence from the waiting room would be more likely to cause speculation around the village, in the bars, the coffee-shops and massage parlours, and among the peasants in the mountains; they'd probably think you weren't well.'

But Joe, in his self-centred narcissistic way, which might in the future qualify him for high political office, did have a point.

'How about this for a plan?' I said. 'Phone me just before your daily visit, I'll leave the rear door unlocked, you can slip in that way and through the back office without anyone noticing, that way only you and I will ever know you've been here, and I shall clasp your secrets to my bosom, even your most sordid little peccadilloes.'

'You and I are of like mind,' said Joe.

'Except,' I said. 'One of us is joking.'

Ask away, but you may not like the answer

GP 20 September 2016

Joe had just received his weekly antibiotic prescription and I was looking forward to a blissful seven Joe-free days when he pulled a piece of paper from his pocket.

'I downloaded this from the NHS Choices website,' he said.

There you go, I thought, even a weakness for online porn can have its Bright Side and can lead to many transferrable and employable skills. Joe might even have a career in the industry; not in front of the camera, of course, Joe never takes his black socks off, which probably disqualifies him.

'According to them, there are a few questions I should ask you,' he continued.

I'm familiar with the website, and the questions, all of which are laudable and beyond reproach and all obviously written by someone who thinks that GPs can spend a fortnight with each patient.

'Ask away,' I said.

'Number 1,' he said. 'Are there other ways to treat my condition?'

'Indeed there are,' I said. 'Almost certainly the best way would be to wait until it gets better on its own. Might take a long time, I admit, maybe 2-3 days.'

Joe shifted in his chair, a bit unhappy with the response.

'Number 2; what do you recommend?'

'That you wait and let it get better on its own.'

Joe could see a pattern emerging, and didn't like the shape.

'Number 3; Is there anything I can do to help myself?'

'Indeed there is,' I said, beginning to enjoy this. 'Stop smoking, take regular exercise, cut down on alcohol, eat a balanced diet, don't run away whenever you see a green vegetable, find a job, move out of your mother's house, generally get a life. Any other questions?'

Joe was more hesitant by now.

'Number 4; do I need to come back and see you?' he read.

'Joe,' I said, 'though it breaks my heart, I must set you free; to paraphrase Jane Austen, you have delighted me long enough.'

An antibiotic, or my left hand?

GP 29 May 2015

Overzealous? Not me. So I knew just what to do when Mrs X told me: 'I've an awful sore throat and I need an antibiotic.'

I'd actually rather cut off my own hand than refuse Mrs X her weekly prescription for antibiotics - it'd save trouble in the long run and probably be less painful. But this time, maybe it'll be different, I thought, maybe we'll work everything out by reason, diplomacy, dialogue and mutual co-operation.

According to the Academy of Medical Royal Colleges (AoMRC), there is growing evidence that pressure for doctors to do something at each consultation has led to patients sometimes receiving treatments that are of little or no value.

Which is hardly news; in ancient Mesopotamia, when he wasn't massacring the neighbours, King Hammurabi was establishing the Code of Hammurabi, one of the earliest surviving codes of law.

Included in this was a law threatening overzealous surgeons with the loss of a hand or an eye. Nowadays, we could just take away their big shiny cars.

'Before I prescribe antibiotics, which of course I shall do with a heart and a half,' I said to Mrs X, 'the good people at AoMRC have advised that you ask me three questions.'

I handed her the list, which she squinted at suspiciously.

'Do I really need this test, procedure, or treatment?' she read.

'No,' I said, 'any more antibiotics and one day a big green monster will jump out of your chest and run screaming down the road.'

Her glare was in the terawatt range, just for me. It made me feel special. 'Are there simpler options?' she continued.

'There certainly are,' I said. 'Heretical though it sounds, medical science would advise rest and plenty of fluids.' This was followed by a long silence, a threatening kind of silence, with shades of a mob, a rope and a hanging.

Finally, she asked: 'What happens if I do nothing?'

'You'll get better on your own,' I said. 'Your immune system, which has evolved over millions of years, will respond to this undoubtedly crippling viral infection with gusto and enthusiasm.'

'That's as may be. I still want an antibiotic,' she said, implacably.

And as the ghost of Hammurabi came whispering to my mind, I thought, well, I don't really need my left hand.

The dark side of being a country doctor

GP 6 January 2016

All the world's a stage, and we docs are but poor players. Mrs Dooley had never attended drama school, but had learned acting from the University of Life, and could teach even the most distinguished thespian about the centrality of the initial visual impact.

As GK Chesterton observed, artifice is the ultimate expression of human genius; things that try to look like things often look more like things than the actual things, and no cripple can have the physical dexterity to be as plausibly crippled as an actor pretending to be a cripple.

Other cripples would point at Mrs Dooley in the street and say, 'Look, isn't she crippled?' She even rather cheered other cripples up – it's always nice to know there's somebody worse off than you.

'The DLA doctor is calling tomorrow,' she said, meaningfully, after her weekly wheezy hobble into the surgery.

Real medicine is the process of making decisions amid diverse influences. It involves discussion, calm deliberation, and the capacity to balance valid but competing interests.

South Armagh is an uncertain country, violently necklaced by a ragged border and long deprived of industry and investment. People have had to learn to live by their wits, which may involve schemes such as smuggling whatever is in this week's hit parade or playing the system like an old Stradivarius.

Mrs Dooley and I had always had a cordial, give-and-take relationship; I gave her what she wanted, and she took it. But this time I was conflicted; there is a Dark Side to being a country doctor. Sometimes we can know our patients a bit too well, and see things we aren't meant to see.

Only the week before I'd witnessed her scamper, gazelle-like, onto the football field to berate an unfortunate referee whose decisions had displeased her.

Should I confront her, I wondered, weighing up my loyalty to the individual patient against the common good of a resource-depleted healthcare system.

I examined my conscience; 'Your options suck,' it told me, helpful as ever.

As so often in medicine, what's right and what's necessary aren't the same thing. The common good and the individual good were in bed together, but individual good had the hot water bottle.

'No problem,' I said. 'You can borrow a wheelchair.'

Every prescription tells a story

GP 12 October 2016

A prescription is much more than just a little piece of paper; it has many fathers - some noble: 'This is to show How Much I Care', some less so: 'This consultation is over, finished, finito, now scram.'

A prescription is convenient, the medical equivalent of handy for the buses and close to the shops. And to the experienced eye, a prescription tells a story, like a great novel, implying much more than is simply written on the page, demanding that the reader employ both imagination and intellect. A prescription is something very special, something to be cherished and valued.

But:

'I lost my fucking prescription,' said Joe.

'I'm sure you don't need a prescription for that,' I said. 'There are more conventional methods; you meet a nice girl, send her flowers, buy her perfume, ask her out, take her to a movie, go dancing, and then, your sturdy yin to her slander yang, who knows what magic the night might bring?'

I was only being partly whimsical; a prescription for sex was probably Joe's best chance as long as he continued to live with his mammy. After all, if we can prescribe exercise, drugs, diets... though I accept it would present a formidable challenge to our pharmacy colleagues.

Joe simply losing his prescription was relatively plausible compared to his usual excuses. Joe's prescriptions seem to be a jinx, a herald of dire calamity for all who dare to approach them.

If a house burns down, Joe's prescription will be in the midst of the inferno. In a multiple-vehicle motorway pile-up, Joe's prescription will inexplicably be sitting on the bonnet. If a rabid dog is on the rampage, the first thing consumed by its slavering jaws will be Joe's prescription.

I must point out that I've never actually observed any of these catastrophes myself; it's what Joe tells me, and is it my job to call him a liar, to be the cold and unattractive hand of reality?

'No,' said Joe, uncertain whether I was being serious or not. 'I actually lost my prescription. Can I have another one?'

If you love something, let it go; if it comes back to you demanding another prescription for antibiotics, you don't want it.

A new year, a new lifestyle; or not...

GP 10 January 2018

As the new year was sinking its ponderous buttocks into the unfortunate armchair of time, Joe again felt ready to take responsibility for his own health. 'I was thinking about changing my ...lifestyle,' he said, clearly struggling with the word, as he did with any health-related issue that didn't involve a prescription.

My clinical instincts are ever alert, and they informed me that Joe had had a curry for breakfast. The stains on his sweat-shirt (which had probably started out life as an ordinary shirt; Joe provided his own sweat) leant strength to this hypothesis.

'Your diet consists of curries and burgers, you take no exercise, you smoke and you drink too much,' I said. 'These violent delights have violent ends.'

Joe belched on cue, a large and pungent punctuation. Food that Joe ate was in trouble; his digestive system did terrible things to food.

'You want me to give up curries and burgers and start taking exercise as well?' he said, 'When sorrows come, they come not single spies. But in battalions!' Our consultation was becoming increasingly Shakespearean.

'Is good health worth being miserable?' his lamentation continued. 'As La Rochefoucauld observed: "To preserve one's health at the cost of too strict a diet is indeed a tedious illness." Anyway, why worry about the future, I've had a good life.'

'Really?' I said, waking up from a Joe-induced stupor for a moment, now genuinely intrigued.

'Some great times,' he said softly, as if still in a post-coital afterglow. 'You remember my STD?'

'It was unforgettable, one of the few things you can't buy on Amazon; yet,' I admitted, considerately leaving out the implied 'you idiot'. 'And also unique, the first person ever to contract an STD without having actual sex with, you know, another person.'

'Those were the days, my friend,' he said sadly.

'I'm not your friend, I'm your doctor,' I said, not wanting any misunderstanding.

'But I'm gonna try anyway,' he said. 'Burgers and curries, they're history.'

I'd heard all this before of course; to paraphrase Dr Johnson, Joe's annual lifestyle change was like a dog shaking hands or poetry in a medical journal.

It wasn't going to be done well, but it was surprising that it was done at all.

When you have nothing more to give

GP 2 February 2016

'The second law of medicine,' I read, disbelievingly, 'no-one cares how much you know till they know how much you care.'

No, seriously, some do-gooder actually wrote that, and it's hard to read without gagging. Next time you're having your prostate examined, look over your shoulder and say, 'You do care, don't you?' I'd want someone dispassionate and clinical, and I'd prefer it not be done in an empathetic and affectionate manner (that's reserved for special friends only, know what I mean?). Glib medical truisms mean nothing.

Nothing.

'Those tablets made me want to vomit,' said Joe, making charming retching noises to emphasis the point.

It was the end of long day, and my usual sunshine disposition had been stunned to muteness by the realisation I was fighting a fundamental law of the universe; Joe would want tablets to correct the vomiting caused by the previous tablets.

The new tablets, in turn, would also cause vomiting, and so on ad infinitum; I was looking at a Dante-esque vision of hell, stretching before me down the ages, an eternity of tales about Joe's vomiting. I was in despair, defeated. I had nothing left, nothing more to offer, nothing I could do for this man.

Nothing.

And then, suddenly, just when the battle seemed lost, I remembered that magical bullshit phrase; 'No-one cares how much you know till they know how much you care.'

'Joe,' I said, affecting a tremor in my voice while clandestinely sticking a needle in my testicles so that genuine tears welled up in my eyes. 'You poor tortured soul; how awful, you've been vomiting, and you kept this all to yourself, fought this battle on your own for, like, three whole days.

'And I know just how you feel,' I continued. 'Brokendown, battered; this week my wife left me for another.'

'Really?' said Joe, fascinated despite his utter self-centredness. 'What was his name?'

'Sally,' I sobbed. 'So you see, I understand your pain; I empathise.'

Amazingly, Joe seemed satisfied that I was even more miserable than him and departed sans prescription, a miraculous and unprecedented state.

Gosh, I thought, if you can fake empathy, you've got it made, I'll have to try this again.

Sometimes Nothing can be a real cool hand.

Looking at you or the computer?

GP 18 January 2016

My friends have come and gone, but Joe seems to have been with me forever, a pungent little black cloud on the horizon. Over the years, admittedly, our relationship has become a little less adversarial; if Joe ever needs an organ donation, he can have my prostate.

And like every beloved enemy, Joe always has some Sunday magazine conceit to whine about.

'You spend all your time looking at your computer instead of me,' he complained.

'Listen buddy,' I said. "First of all, you're no oil-painting, though I accept that you have a certain Rubenesque quality.'

'But my body is a temple,' he said.

'Sure it is,' I agreed. 'A big fat hairy temple.'

'Secondly,' I continued. 'To input the precious information you disclose, I must look at the computer; I have to click this goddam mouse about a thousand times for each patient. But a demonstration is worth a thousand words; so tell me, why you are here today?'

'I have an awful pain in my arm,' said Joe, then added (as is obligatory) 'It's awful bad, I've been fighting it all week.'

'OK,' I said. 'I shall now attempt to type that in without looking at the computer, to try to express how much you are suffering, whilst all the time staring into your baby-blue eyes.'

I then invited Joe to inspect the results, preserved for all eternity in his Electronic Health Record (which I understand is somewhere up there in The Cloud).

In accordance with the rules of universal humour, it read, 'Awful pain in the arse.'

Changing lifestyle? There's an easier way

GP 17 May 2016

'If liberty means anything at all, it means the right to tell people what they do not want to hear,' said George Orwell.

So; 'I think you should consider changing your lifestyle, Joe,' I ventured.

'Life-style,' he said, pronouncing the word slowly, drawing it out, savouring it as if it was some rare new sweet, but one with a nasty after-taste.

'You know, exercise and all,' I explained, patient education always my priority. Joe looked around, as if sensing a trap closing in, and to my surprise, began to smite me with cunning arguments.

'Let's not rush into anything, doc,' he said. 'Pills get a bad rap, but they're perfect for use in the home, like when you're sitting on the sofa watching Sky Sports.

'But a good walk and five portions of fresh fruit or vegetables every day would be as good as any pill,' I said.

'Yeh,' said Joe. 'And I could heed the call of the wolf and hunt for myself as well, rejoice in the thrill of the chase and exult as I slake my thirst on the fresh warm blood of my new-slaughtered prey.

'But it's a damn sight more convenient when my mammy sticks it on a plate in front of me.'

Homoerotic? No thanks

GP 27 June 2017

'Dr X is no good,' said Joe.

I know Dr X well, a fine chap, and a trusted colleague, but it's always a relief to know that some other poor sod will be finding a cow's head at the bottom of his bed (the Irish version of a mafia threat).

In medicine there's always a choice. I first considered appeasement - give Joe the antibiotics/sleeping tablets/vitamins, i.e. chicken out; and anyway, patient care is being replaced by customer satisfaction, isn't it?

But that would be disloyal to my colleague, and even worse, encourage Joe's help-seeking behaviour and mark me down as a soft touch.

And during every surgery there is something to be won.

Joe coughed loudly, in the way only some with a perfectly functioning respiratory system could cough; I've had sex which was less vigorous and required less physical dexterity.

'Antibiotics,' I explained, 'are like F-words. One or two is fine. Forty-five is bad.'

Joe coughed again, more expressively this time. A bodily function is worth a thousand words.

'Delayed gratification is so often the key to success,' I continued. 'Someday you will really need an antibiotic, and eschewing it today may mean it will save your life then. As Holly Johnson sang, 'Relax, don't do it/When you wanna go to it.' Okay, that came out a little more homoerotic than I intended.'

'Homoerotic,' said Joe suspiciously, as if the word was some new and foreign dessert. 'If it's homoerotic I don't want it.'

Result, I thought.

A painful experience

GP 31 May 2017

I must be modest here, as I was once described as a beautiful young man with the body of a Greek God (admittedly, this was by my Auntie Mamie, some Irish families are a bit odd).

So when Joe arrive with a big bandage across his fore-head I was impressed by the rakish, piratical and rather dashing effect.

'Head wounds clearly suit you,' I said.

'I tripped over the dog,' he said.

'And has your dog ever done this before?' I asked shrewdly; the experienced clinician always takes a careful past medical history.

'I don't know,' he dead-panned. 'It wasn't my dog.'

As I have a compassionate, humanitarian side, I un-wrapped the bandage. The abrasion was disappointingly small. I replaced Bandage-zilla with a teeny-weeny sticking plaster, just to show How Much I Care. Joe gave a satisfying little yelp.

'That hurt,' he said.

I am always alert to the responsibilities of our profession; though preventive medicine may seem less than heroic, it forms an important part of the consultation.

'Pain is a teacher, a guide, a learning experience,' I told him. 'One that is always there to both warn us of our limitations and challenge us to overcome them.

'For something no one likes, pain does us a whole hell of a lot of good. Everything important that will ever happen to us in life is going to involve pain to one degree or another; as Shakespeare said, 'Pain pays the income of each precious thing'. It rips away our vanities and confusions, helps us remember that life is about loving and being loved, about living in the now and accepting the simple joys of the beauty of the world.

'Some people say that pain is our greatest friend; mind you, some people will say anything.'

The passing of the sceptre

GP 10 July 2015

I've never lost my reverence for good colleagues, those warriors who battle ceaselessly against the dark, on the side of the angels, even if the angels don't like it very much.

The average age of a patient in general practice is 75; multiple diagnoses, incredibly complex care, increased expectations and ever-reducing resources, but as Epictetus said: 'The greater the difficulty, the more glory in surmounting it; skilful pilots earn their reputation from storms and tempests.'

Like Tennyson's Ulysses, we have drunk the delight of battle. But there comes a time when we're no longer that strength which in old days moved earth and heaven, and we must pass on our values of sacrifice and selfless dedication.

'I don't like going to see doctors,' said Joe.

'And doctors don't like you going to see doctors either,' I agreed, glad we had found some common ground, building a relationship, although maybe not quite ready to start dating yet.

'Look at this,' he said.

It was scary, but then I had a brainwave; I have a degree, you know (and diplomas, which don't really count – Diploma of Child Health, Diploma in Obstetrics, just pay the exorbitant fee and they throw the scroll at you).

The registrar should see this, I thought, he needs the experience. 'Have you examined it?' he asked me, with puppy-like naivety, clearly wondering if the college had a protocol for this kind of thing.

'What do you think, my Telemachus?' I answered – because the open-ended response encourages the registrar to think for himself.

'We'd better examine it,' he said.

'If you want to get that close, be my guest,' I said. 'I'll be observing you from far away, with a telescope.' I passed him the rubber gloves, but before I could shout a warning, he poked at the unexploded sebaceous cyst, with catastrophic consequences.

'Smells like something died in here,' said Joe.

Complimentary medicine

GP 20 October 2015

Joe is always grumpy, that diplomatic post at the United Nations getting further and further away every day. I have to admit, he's very good at it, and there is a bright side; when he leaves the surgery, there's an immediate lightening of the spirit, a sense of freedom and relief, like the sun coming out from behind a cloud on a winter's day, or Liverpool getting a manager who actually knows what he's doing, or the passing of a well-formed bowel movement after a prolonged episode of constipation.

So it was rather disconcerting when he came in one day beaming and showering me with compliments. I had good reason to be wary; compliments can be double-edged and manipulative, and the wise clinician will look for an ulterior motive. As William Wilberforce said: 'Flatterers are not your friends; nay sir, they are your deadliest enemies.'

Everyone likes a bit of approval. Fire out sick certs and sleeping tablets and antibiotics on request, refer every headache for a brain scan, and you'll be everybody's best buddy.

But patients aren't your buddy; their expectations and what we consider to be in their best interests often come into conflict.

We don't strive to give patients what they want, but what they need. We husband precious resources, and the hardest part of medicine is knowing when not to use it. It's not a doctor's job to be popular, and it's much more important that we like our patients than that they like us.

'We were talking about you last night at the match; nobody had a bad word to say about you,' said Joe, 'And anybody that did, I soon put them right.'

There was some ambiguity to this compliment, but I accepted it gracefully.

'Thanks for your support, Joe,' I said, 'But you're still not getting any antibiotics.'

Consumer receptive alternative preparations (CRAP)

BMJ 12 May 2010

Joe was a veritable cornucopia of symptoms and a technicolour array of risk factors, and I looked out the window in the despairing hope that the clouds might form themselves into a plausible diagnosis. They did their best, amusingly shaping themselves into a pair of rather ripe and Rubenesque buttocks that might have put even a post-therapy Tiger Woods off his swing, but I had just about given up when a bus rolled by with a big advert on the side, and I stood like stout Cortez, silent upon a peak on Darién.

Aristotle and Spinoza believed that all human behaviour is self-referential, and boy were they right. I was being selfish; I had kept Joe all to myself, it was time for generosity, time to share.

'Have you considered trying a health food shop?' I asked.

'I heard they sold crap,' he said.

'Perhaps,' I said, 'but not just any old CRAP, it's brightly coloured, attractively packaged CRAP. Even better, according to the ads, it's half price CRAP.'

'I note,' said Joe perspicaciously, 'that the word 'CRAP' is a recurring theme; you have used it three times already.'

'What I tell you three times is true,' I protested.

'Presenting Carrollian nonsense instead of a solid evidence base is not a persuasive argument,' said Joe.

'Look,' I said, not giving up, 'Go into any high street pharmacy and you will see row upon row of homeopathic preparations, vitamin and mineral supplements, and flower remedies, some of them used for thousands of years by a rainforest tribe who survive on a diet of honeydew and possum sweat. Now remember, because this is important: pharmacists are highly trained healthcare professionals, and surely it would be against their ethical code to stock and thereby give implicit approval to treatments that have not been proved to be effective.'

'And yet,' said Joe, refusing to display an open mind, 'the pharmacists claim that there is a consumer demand for these products. So they stock homeopathic products purely because they sell, not because they work.'

'But you can't overdose, and they're very safe,' I tried one last time.

'Yes,' Joe admitted grudgingly, 'You can't have too much CRAP.'

Want a friend? Get a dog

BMJ 3 August 2011

'I have a list,' said Joe. As inflammatory opening gambits go, it's hard to beat.

Osler advised equanimity as the second most important medical virtue, next to sarcasm. So over many years I have cultivated a tranquil demeanour, which the casual observer might misinterpret as apathy. I sat back in my chair, closed my eyes, counted to ten, let peace come dropping slow upon linnet's wings; a mote of dust floated down.

Accordingly, my response was a study in restraint.

'Take your list and get the f*** out of here,' I said. 'What do you think this is? A supermarket?'

'Calm down, calm down,' said Joe, in what I had to grudgingly admit was a passable imitation of Harry Enfield; the needle of humour can puncture and deflate even the most promising argument.

'I have only two items,' he explained, 'Firstly, I want to be detoxified.'

'Words are plastic,' I said. 'Terrorists become insurgents; innocent victims become civilian casualties before morphing into collateral damage; Bono is an international philanthropist rather than a greedy tax dodger; and detoxification is no longer the process by which toxins are changed into less toxic or more readily excretable substances but instead a callous pseudoscience that allows the fleecing of vulnerable punters by avaricious charlatans.

'There you are,' I continued, googling 'detoxification' and skipping over the inevitable pages of celebrities. 'Detox diets, detox recipes, detox tea, detox footpads (for those of us who wish to excrete urea through our feet), and detox plutonium. Apparently, any old rubbish can be flogged simply by putting the word 'detox' in front of it. It's the timeless *pas de deux* of gullibility and greed.'

'OK, OK, it's a crock, I get it,' he said. 'Only a complete idiot would fall for it.'

'You'd have to be a real sucker,' I agreed, secretly astounded that logic had, for once, proved to be helpful during a consultation. 'And your second item?'

'I added you as a friend on Facebook,' he accused, 'and you haven't answered.' Social media are perilous; becoming overly chummy may corrode our mystique and degrade our relationship with lay people.

'Let's think about detox again,' I said.

Run wild, run free

BMJ 7 May 2013

When Joe hangs his coat on the hook it's a territorial marker, like a hyena widdling on a tree.

'I'm here,' it says, 'And I'm here for a while, till I'm ready to go, and nobody is gonna shift me.'

His style looked preppie, with just a hint of old Etonian. Charming bits and bobs fell out during the process, from which the astute clinician could garner information about the patient's lifestyle: pipes, used bookies' dockets (retained in case the race is miraculously run again), ancient tissues. His clothes were an autobiography: 'Through tattered clothes great vices do appear.'

Frayed jockeys off, and there he was—naked. Hold your friends close, and your enemies closer, said Sun Tzu in *The Art of War*, and I have always held Joe very closely indeed, so close that, most of the time, I'm actually behind him; on aesthetic grounds this is the preferred point of view, especially when Joe is (pre-examination) naked.

But strangely, no matter how many clothes Joe took off, he never seemed completely naked, because Joe is a hairy man. A really hairy man. So hairy that when he is naked you can't tell he is naked. A hundred years ago he'd have been in a sideshow tent and charging a fee. Venturing a stethoscope in there was like Stanley plunging headlong through the Congo rainforest, and just as sweaty.

It may sound repulsive, but experience has taught me how to surmount this. Joe is like a pet, and he has everything a pet should have—that is, a glossy coat, bright eyes, sweet breath, and the whitest teeth. Added to all these, he has the charm of speech and reason. Nothing could be more disgusting than the one impression; nothing more delightful than the other. It all depends on the point of view.

'Run wild, mighty stallion,' I said, 'and glory in the wind blowing freely through your bodily orifices.'

I opened the door and set him free.

I heard screams outside.

'Good night, sweet prince,' I said, 'May flights of angels sing thee to thy rest. And you forgot your jockeys.'

Beware the Friend

GP 5 November 2009

'Can I bring a Friend in?' said Mrs Murphy, a shy and self-effacing lady.

'Of course,' I said grandly, suspecting a 'woman's problem', but when the Friend entered the surgery I knew I had made a big mistake.

The Friend was a large lady with an unmistakeable air of menace. But hark! The cry is Astur, I thought; the room seemed to immediately shrink and become uncomfortably warm. The Friend nodded to me and there was something in the gesture which implied it wasn't a million miles from a head butt.

'I've been having trouble sleeping,' began Mrs Murphy. 'It's been going on for some time now. I toss and turn all night and I'm exhausted in the morn... '

'She needs sleeping tablets,' interrupted the Friend.

'I see,' I said. 'Perhaps, Mrs Murphy, you could tell me a little more. For example, do you have a nap during the day... '

'She needs sleeping tablets,' said the Friend, cracking her knuckles meaningfully.

'There are many methods of improving your sleeping pattern,' I said, all the time aware of the Friend's gimlet gaze, and desperately trying to maintain eye contact with Mrs Murphy, who had by this stage relinquished all executive authority over her own person.

'It's important to take plenty of exercise, avoid naps during the day and coffee and tea late at...'

'She needs sleeping tablets,' said the Friend, implacable.

'Sleeping tablets are not to be prescribed lightly,' I said, trying to lighten the mood and give things that personal touch. 'And if you were my mother or,' here I gave the Friend what I hoped was a winning smile, 'a youthful auntie, and a doctor prescribed you sleeping tablets, I wouldn't be very happy.'

'So you wouldn't give your mother a prescription,' said the Friend coldly.

'Sleeping tablets have many unwanted effects,' I tried to explain, fingering the panic button...

'Listen,' said the Friend, 'she ain't your mother and I sure ain't your auntie.' And I'll kick the shit out of you in a minute, she implied.

'A short course of nitrazepan will help,' I agreed, surrendering.

As Muhammed Ali said, 'He who fights and runs away/Lives to fight another day.'

The use and abuse of reverse psychology

GP 12 November 2009

We are come to the waning of the year, and a familiar refrain will echo across the land and through the surgeries. Like the sound of wild geese honking triumphantly as they spiral down the wind over the Mourne Mountains to Carlingford Lough, wild wings from the northlands returning to the country of Finn and Oisin, landing in a rush and whirl of freezing spray, dawn's early light glinting coldly on their silver-grey feathers.

'My Auntie Allie got the flu jab, and she was sick for a month after,' said Joe defiantly, like generations before him; some traditions defy the years.

'Slow though I am to impugn the veracity of your Auntie Allie,' I said, 'even if it be the same Auntie Allie who claimed to have fought at the Alamo and been Davy Crockett's secret concubine, all the evidence suggests that the flu vaccine is both protective against the flu and very safe.'

'I still don't want it,' he insisted stoutly, which meant it was time for a bit of reverse psychology.

'That's great,' I said. 'It'll save us a fortune, the vaccine is very expensive, you know, which is why we only give it to selected individuals.

'Did I tell you I'm thinking of buying a new car? A big shiny car, with all the bells on, the make doesn't matter, so long as it's big and shiny.'

'Expensive, is it?' said Joe, 'So that's the reason you don't want me to have it. I want that jab.'

'Oh alright, if you absolutely insist,' I said, whipping out a syringe and slipping it into his arm before he could have second thoughts.

'And can you guarantee that it's perfectly safe?' he asked, rubbing his arm gingerly.

This is a dilemma we must frequently confront. To treat our patients as mature adults we must share our reservations that no treatment is perfectly safe, nor is it guaranteed to work; in the real world, shit happens. Unfortunately, in doing this we lose the placebo effect and cede ground to the charlatans of complementary medicine.

'If you want guarantees, go to a bank,' I replied, 'Not an Irish bank, of course.'

You can't teach an old hypochondriac new tricks

GP 3 October 2012

The years had not been kind to Joe.

He came from a broken home (a JCB had crashed into his house), and his mother would come in with him to the surgery until he was in his early twenties.

Like all Irish mothers, she managed to be both soothing and reassuring yet frightening and intimidating all at the same time, and if that was her effect on me, what was it like for Joe? He was so complicated he should have come with a manual.

A chubby chap, like Oliver Hardy (without the sense of humour), he was a firm subscriber to Dylan Thomas's philosophy: 'Do not go gentle into that good night/Rage, rage against the dying of the light,' but decided to so subscribe at an inappropriately early age.

Every symptom was a cause of immediate and bitter anguish but also a harbinger of disaster further down the line. Optimism, he believed, was the result of intellectual error; *timor mortis conturbat me* might have been his motto.

His one release was his interest in Gaelic football. In Crossmaglen, we are fortunate to have a mighty team, with innumerable county titles and a few All-Ireland championships. But even this interest was coloured by his implacable pessimism, allowing him to be always armoured against defeat and alert for disappointment.

'That'll be no good against the Kerry and Cork teams,' he'd opine, after we hoovered up yet another Ulster title. Even if we were 20 points ahead, when the opposition broke briefly upfield he'd say, 'I told you this would happen,' in a doom-laden tone.

And if they managed a consolation score, 'Ah, we're bate now,' shaking his head sadly, like a fat Irish Cassandra prophesying ruin before the gates of Troy. Winning the All-Ireland entailed no joy, no living in the moment, just visions of a bleak future: 'That's the last one.'

Nonetheless, because I am sometimes a good doctor, I somehow persuaded Joe to take up regular exercise and less than a year later, he completed his first marathon, in under four hours.

'That was brilliant, Joe,' I said, hoping that a surge of endorphins would have modified his brain chemistry.

'My feet are killing me,' he said.

The Curse of the Irish Mammy

GP 12 October 2010

I always expect the worst. In fact, if the worst doesn't happen, I'm a bit disappointed, and also apprehensive; it's not that the worst hasn't happened, just that it hasn't happened yet.

Near the end of the surgery, I was feeling good. It had been a fulfilling day; a few challenging diagnoses, a couple of moral conundrums, the patients and I relating well and working together in a true sense of partnership and all that shite. I felt good, I had helped some people, brought a little light into the world, done the state some service.

But because I felt good, I felt bad. I knew it couldn't last, the universe would once again conspire against me. So it was with a sense of fatal satisfaction that I watched Joe trudge morosely into the room; the balance of the cosmos had returned, all was in equilibrium again.

'Those tablets were no good,' he said.

'As I have told you many times before, Joe,' I said wearily, 'There is no such thing as a tablet that will make you more attractive to women.'

'They were useless,' said Joe doggedly.

I considered despair yet rejected it utterly; there's a little Don Quixote in every family doctor; that our deeds prove to be futile makes them no less valiant.

'Because I care so much,' I said, 'And also because I am at my wit's end, I am going to suggest something revolutionary yet academically impeccable.'

'What's that?' said Joe, suspiciously.

'Lifestyle, Joe,' I said, 'you need to change your lifestyle. Start exercising, lose weight, take a night course, get a job.'

To my surprise, Joe seemed to be actually listening.

'I could do that,' he said, a determined expression appearing on his face; a determined expression requires more effort than a bored expression, so looked quite disorienting on Joe.

I pinched myself, wondering if I was hallucinating.

'Anything else?' he asked.

'Stop smoking, drink in moderation, find a rewarding hobby, cultivate a sunny disposition.'

'Yes,' he said enthusiastically, 'I can change, it's time for a new me, the old Joe is dead, let's go for it.'

'Just one thing,' I said, 'you'll have move out of your mammy's house; otherwise you'll always look like a total loser.'

'Could we try another tablet?' he said.

Defeated yet defiant

BMJ 22 May 2008

'Hurrah for Captain Spaulding,' I carolled as the door opened, which I thought quite droll, because his name, can you believe it, was Joe Spaulding. But the infectious bonhomie of Groucho Marx proved no defence against the horror that was to come; Joe was turning his back and pulling down his trousers even before the door was shut.

'Hold it right there, pal,' I said—but it was too late. I had no shotgun, and the cattle prod was on the blink.

'What do you think?' he asked.

This was an ambiguous question. I considered and rejected 'You have beautiful soft skin' and 'Look at those fine taut muscles—have you been working out?' before finally settling on, 'I think I wish I was a thousand miles away, lying on a beach with a young lady massaging aromatic oils into my rippling muscles.' I'm not totally opposed to complementary medicine.

But this was the incorrect response, and Joe started to reverse, inch by dreadful inch. Denial is a powerful mechanism, but I could deny it no longer: Joe wanted me to peer closely and intimately between his buttocks.

I have always had a sensitive disposition. I don't like actual physical contact (except when it involves certain types of complementary medicine). I don't like touching patients; you never know where they've been. Anyway, this physical examination stuff is overrated. It's for theatrical purposes only (to show How Much We Care). I'm a great believer in the primacy of the history.

'I've this awful rash,' the bare cheeks mimed, edging ever closer.

I retreated, but the cheeks kept coming. I emptied the sharps box, but the massive quivering buttocks ground inexorably closer, and the little needles lay squashed and pathetic, like Trojans on the banks of the Scamander as Achilles turned the river red.

I shrank back into a corner, a wild animal at bay.

'Alright, alright,' I sobbed, 'I see it, I see it, it's a rash, a rash.'

'What kind of rash?'

'An awful rash. Oh God, it's awful. I'll give you some cream.'

'And?' The buttocks wobbled threateningly, by now right in my face.

'Antibiotics—you need antibiotics,' I screamed, frantically scribbling on a prescription pad with averted eyes. And as a drowsy numbness pained my sense, with a final defiant gesture I signed it 'Hugo Z Hackenbush.'

The man and the orifice

GP 17 October 2007

'These young junior doctors,' said Joe. 'They're so full of energy, so passionate, so enthusiastic, so idealistic. How is it then that they all turn into fat complacent consultants who only ambition in life is a big shiny car and a reserved parking spot. Is it like that Kafka novel, Metamorphosis, where a man wakes up one day as a cockroach?'

'You are utterly mistaken Joe,' I said, momentarily discommoded by Joe's unexpected display of literary scholarship.

'Your image of consultants is completely based on the Sir Lancelot Spratt caricature. I admit that some of the noxious breed may still exist in dark corners, usually identified by the word emeritus, but I assure you that all the consultants I know are hard-working, diligent, and deeply committed to the NHS, yet under more and more pressure each day from increased expectations, reduced resources and ever-expanding bureaucracy.'

'But that last one you sent me to,' said Joe. 'He wasn't very nice.'

'Alas,' I said. 'Being nice to you is not in his job specification; being nice to you is one of the many bucks that stop with me. It can be an onerous burden, but one that fate has ordained I must carry alone.'

'He hardly spoke a word to me,' said Joe, as his voice took on a rather offended and embarrassed tone, 'And when he examined me, he was very……. rough.'

'Rough?' I enquired.

'Rough compared to you, I mean,' said Joe. 'You were very gentle, more …sensitive.'

'Ah, indeed', I said, 'But then my sensitivity to the more delicate parts of the male anatomy is by now legendary; the peasants in the mountains sing a folk song about it.'

I shuddered; I'd repressed the memory of exploring the Congo of Joe's body. Repression is how we Irish deal with things, and it's all the fault of the British, Before you invaded we were a bawdy, uninhibited, licentious folk, but you left us a crippling legacy of Victorian prudery (especially regarding sex).

What Joe had interpreted as 'gentleness' had instead been a cocktail of fear, timidity and revulsion. 'My God,' I remembered thinking (there are no atheists in foxholes). 'I am going to have to actually, like, touch him.'

142

And now the memories came flooding back as my subconscious gave up the unequal struggle; inside I was screaming like a little girl.

'I'm not going back to him, I don't care what he says,' said Joe, stubbornness to the point of constipation being considered a virtue among Ireland's stout yeomanry.

'According to this letter, Joe', I said, 'your prostate is like a grapefruit, albeit without the beguiling citrus aroma. It further says that you will need an operation which may greatly relieve your unpleasant symptoms.'

'I'm not going back.'

'Okay, I can't twist your arm, you can carry on dribbling like a dysfunctional mannequin pis de Bruxelles and getting up to pee more times each night than Ronaldo will dive in a season, it's your call.'

'He'll have to apologise first,' said Joe.

'There are two chances of that. Slim and none, and Slim is in a private hospital in Grenada having a hernia repair on the cheap.'

I really wanted Joe to have the surgery, partly for his own well-being and partly because I didn't want him torturing me about his nocturnal afflictions for the next cajillion years.

It was time for a desperate gamble.

'The surgeon doesn't care whether you turn up or not,' I said. 'To him you are just another orifice, one among thousands he is compelled to inspect each week. But to me you are much more than that.' Here I paused for a long moment. 'You are a patient and a... friend.'

Joe looked a bit surprised, our relationship had previously been rather adversarial, in a mutually satisfying way.

'Well, if you feel that way about it, I may as well go ahead,' he said.

'Great,' I said ostentatiously pressing the buzzer for the next patient.

My new friend turned at the door.

'Me and the lads are going fishing tonight, would you like to come along?' he asked, tentatively exploring the boundaries of this new chumminess.

'Fat chance,' I said.

Torture; the bright side (1)

BMJ 17 November 2010

'She preferred the timid touchings of the eunuch to the ponderous bollocks of the Roman Emperor,' said Gibbon's *Decline and Fall of the Roman Empire*, a metaphor for the empire's descent from barbarian virility to effete decadence.

And we are learning nothing from history, because MI6 recently admitted that it regards torture as illegal and abhorrent, and I've been left yearning for those golden days of redneck vigour and bigotry, when *Ad extirpanda*, a papal bull promulgated in 1252, authorised the use of torture by the Inquisition, and when George Bush approved waterboarding.

But despite Pope Innocent and Dubya being cool with it, torture gets a bad rap from the liberal media. The term itself is pejorative, and I prefer 'inhuman and degrading treatment,' as suggested by the European Court of Human Rights.

One method, used in Guantanamo Bay, involved putting prisoners in a box with an insect—after first reassuring them that the insect had neither a venomous sting nor bite. I'll bet the terrorists were shaking in their shoes: 'Please don't throw me in that briar patch, Br'er Fox,' they'd be singing. Could there be a more instructive symbol of the feebleness of the West?

If it was up to Barack Hussein Obama, when the terrorists attack we'll all be sitting around in a circle, holding hands, and singing *Kum bay ya*. The Yanks could learn from the British Army; those chaps know a thing or two about extracting enthusiastic confessions.

Joe told me how, during the Troubles, when they were imprisoning people for the suspicious crime of being called Paddy or Seamus, the army blindfolded him, took him up in a helicopter, then pitched him out. Only when he landed did he realise that the helicopter had lifted just a few feet off the ground. He sprained his left pinky and was lame for hours and hours, another Martyr for Old Ireland.

'That was real torture,' he said, misty-eyed. 'We might have been enemies but, dammit, we respected each other, more substance in our enmity than in our love.' Taking a degree was quite de rigueur among the internees. Joe had read English lit and never flinched from displaying his scholarship. 'You'd have told them anything, just to see their smile; great people, the British.

'But those were hard times,' he added. 'The memories haunt me at night, the world more full of weeping than you can understand.'

'You're still not getting any sleeping tablets,' I said.

Footnote; Torture is now to be described as *enhanced interrogation.*

Torture; the bright side (2)

BMJ 16 Jun 2011

The traditional consultation is a dinosaur; to be fit for purpose, it must adapt to an ever-changing world. But until now our hands have been tied, because the doctor-patient relationship is unequal. Patients can lie to our faces, while we are expected to be honest and truthful; it's like a medical dhimmitude. Well, I'm mad as hell and I'm not gonna take it anymore.

'Honestly, doc,' said Joe smugly, unaware of my new arrangements, 'I don't smoke.'

'Joe,' I said, giving him one last chance, 'Your fingers and teeth are stained the colour of horse manure and your breath would asphyxiate a hyena. I'm asking you again; do you smoke?'

'Not one puff,' he said defiantly.

The gauntlet had been thrown down, so dauntless the slughorn to my lips I set, and two burly colonels marched in.

'These gentlemen are from the US embassy,' I said.

'I don't believe it,' said Joe, 'Let me see your badges.'

'Badges? We don't need no steenking badges,' they said, setting exactly the right tone. They grabbed Joe, pushing him back on the couch. I produced a rag and a large jug of water, placed the rag over his mouth and started pouring.

'Water-boarding is of ancient provenance,' I said conversationally, the sound of gagging an almost musical counterpoint, 'It was first used by the Inquisition, you know, those Catholics could teach us a thing or two. Water-boarding, sounds quite nice, doesn't it, rather refreshing, like a mountain stream, like surf-boarding; goes to show,

146

names can be misleading. A rose by any other name would smell as sweet, I don't think so. Now, once again, do you smoke?'

'Alright, alright,' he sobbed, after exactly 17 secs (thereby lasting longer than Christopher Hitchens or the average CIA operative), 'I confess, I smoke like a train, and by the way, care assistants aren't being adequately trained, Donald Trump's hair is fake, and Bin Laden is in Pakistan, check out the big house in Abbottabad with all the barbed wire, he'll be hiding in the bedroom.'

The colonels stood Joe up, saluted smartly and left, administering one last hefty kick in the kidneys in a graceful American gesture of farewell.

'This is an outrage,' he said, shaken and white-faced, 'That was torture.'

'I'm re-branding it, Joe,' I said, 'That was *enhanced* consultation.'

Cough it up, my son

GP 16 October 2009

'How long have you had this cough?' I enquired, because I am sometimes a Good Doctor, and I like to be thorough.

'Oh, for a good while now,' replied Joe, which was not very informative, I thought.

'Are you bringing up any phlegm?' I asked (being systematic is one of my two great clinical virtues, the others being apathy and vindictiveness, my three great clinical virtues).

'Yeah, buckets of the stuff,' he enthused.

'And what colour is it?'

He looked at me as if I had just arrived from another (more hygienic) dimension.

'What do you mean?' he asked, palpably mystified.

'Well,' I said slowly, 'when you spit it out on a hanky, is it green or yellow, or is it clear and watery, like a waterfall in the rain-forest, where the dolphins play and all the people live in harmony with nature?'

He shook his head firmly, quite unmoved by the haunting imagery I had so carefully crafted. 'I never spit it out,' he said.

'So, you just swallow these buckets of phlegm you have alluded to,' I said.

'You are implying,' he said, wonderingly, 'that I should be laying it out for inspection. I'll admit, that had never occurred to me.'

'You aren't a doctor, how could you have known,' I reassured him.

'But I like to be helpful,' he said, and began to expectorate loudly. I had to hand it to him, he was really trying, doing his best, giving it loads, and it sounded like a horse being strangled.

'Go on, my son,' I said encouragingly.

The phone rang.

'Is everything all right in there?' enquired the receptionist, 'It's just that a crowd has gathered, and there is a rumour going round that you are torturing someone.'

By this stage Joe was blue in the face, and gagging. He gestured frantically, and I passed him a specimen jar, into which he deposited the fruit of his labours.

We looked at it in a contemplative silence.

Eventually: 'A rather disappointing result, I think,' I observed sadly.

'Yeah,' he said defensively, 'but it's green, ain't it? That's gotta count for something.'

'Wins you an antibiotic,' I said.

The sentinel

BMJ 16 November 2011

The hordes are out there, just outside the surgery door. Because freedom isn't free; the price is eternal vigilance, yet, demeaningly, we are called 'gatekeepers' by those we protect, as if we are standing at a booth handing out tickets.

'I've an awful cough and an awful sore throat,' said Joe, 'and I've been fighting it all week.' I checked to see if I had a military cross handy and if the Queen was available for the presentation ceremony.

'And 'they' said I should get some antibiotics.'

They again, I thought, the hydra-headed enemy, the barbarian at the gates.

'Earth has not anything to show more fair,' said William Wordsworth, 'than a big pair of swollen pus covered tonsils.' It's always a welcome sight to us general practitioners because it means we can fire ahead and prescribe antibiotics with a clear conscience and avoid yet another draining fight.

But Joe's throat, predictably, was absolutely completely positively normal—not a speck of pus, not a fleck of erythema. Even the soaring imagination of Arthur C Clarke would have shrivelled in the face of such unflinching normality.

But the war against unreason and wasted resources is unending. Ours is a thankless duty, yet no less noble for that. If a deed is valiant and brave, does it matter that the minstrels do not make a song of it?

Yet we do not begrudge them their innocence and ignorance. General practitioners don't brag of ourselves. We don't have flags or old school songs or *esprit de corps*; we don't wear robes or hoods; we don't do academic processions or gaudy pageantry. We don't need these superficial things because our cause is just, and our bonds run deep; for us, every day is St Crispin's Day. We are the few, the happy few, we band of brothers.

'It's a virus,' I said.

Aliens

GP 11 May 2008

There are some advantages to the unbearable *ennui* of family practice. Nothing surprises us anymore, and we retain our equanimity even in the face of the bizarre and the perverse.

If Jesus himself was to walk into my surgery, I'd probably say, 'Yea, Lord, smite the unbeliever and all, could I have your address and date of birth, please?', and tap in a computer code for 'Visited by Our Saviour.'

So when Mrs Magee came in with Sharon and announced that they had been abducted by aliens, I wasn't a bit fazed.

'And when did this happen?' I asked, pretending to be interested, although yawning hugely does tend to give the game away

'Just yesterday, after Neighbours,' she said, 'A big spaceship landed bedside the house, these insect-like creatures with big teeth came rushing out, killed all the menfolk and wrecked the house, though thankfully the TV was OK.'

'They carried me and our Sharon into their ship and set us down beside these big, pod-shaped things. The pods opened and two horrible spidery creatures jumped on our faces. My one gave up almost immediately and started to throw up, don't know why that happened. When they were all busy giving the sick one a nebuliser, I pulled the other one off our Sharon's face and we ran for it.'

I wasn't inclined to believe this incredible story at first, but when I looked closely at Sharon, she had marks on her face that were consistent with, even diagnostic of, al- iens grabbing at chubby cheeks, and a distended (more than usual) abdomen.

I'd seen the film, and knew what was coming next, but not in my surgery, I thought, all that mess, blood and guts everywhere, who's gonna clean up? What are A&E de- partments for, anyway?

'This is very serious, Mrs Magee,' I said gravely, 'Sharon is the victim of an alien infestation. You will note her distended abdomen, at any moment an alien parasite is going to burst out of there quicker than England from the World Cup. You must take her to Casualty at once; and bring a mop.'

'Thank goodness,' she said, sounding relieved, 'I was worried it was a case of teenage obesity.'

What does the patient want?

BMJ 27 November 2003

"What made you suspicious, Farrell?"

Holmes was a trifle unimaginative, but he was a stout fellow and well worth his keep, as the big problem with a meritocracy is that good servants are hard to find; when everybody's somebody, then nobody's anybody.

"It was the curious incident of the cough in the night," I said.

"But the patient did not cough in the night," said Holmes.

"Exactly," I said, "and that was the curious incident."

A symptom's absence may sometimes be as telling as its presence. Joe was an almost daily attender, could never leave without a prescription, and had as many symptoms as there are stars in the sky, so when he said he had yet another headache I was not overly concerned. He had nausea and vomiting, yet was the headache worse in the morning and on leaning forward? Of course. Had he double vision? No.

And I heard a cock crow three times. For Joe to deny a symptom was as rare as somebody who declares war and actually takes part in it.

After 20 years in practice, I'm hard to shock, so I was only mildly surprised when Joe's skin suddenly turned a bilious green, his ears grew longer and even hairier, and antennae sprouted from his head, all of which actually improved his appearance.

"I am an emissary from the planet Zarg," he said, his voice sibilant and his breath pungent yet noxious, his forked tongue dripping acid saliva on my foot. "Our beloved Emperor Peebo has been most gravely ill for many years and I have long been seeking a physician both wise and intuitive who might provide a cure for this distressing malady. If you succeed you shall be deemed Lord of all Doctors in the Universe and our two peoples shall abide in everlasting friendship."

"What are his Majesty's symptoms?" I asked.

"He has a sore throat and has been bringing up horrible green phlegm."

"Gosh, Joe," I said, "the things you'll do to get an antibiotic."

Sputum clear as a mountain stream...

GP 19 April 2016

If coughs were conductors, Joe would be Daniel Barenboim. He has a whole orchestra at his disposal, from whiny and high-pitched, like the piccolo, to a deep and sonorous, like the double bass.

Joe is also alert to every literary device; in rhetoric, an *epizeuxis* is the repetition of a word or phrase in immediate succession, typically within the same sentence, for vehemence or emphasis. Employing his own unique medical variant of an epizeuxis, Joe coughed twice, just to show he could, looking very smug and pleased with himself – and judging from the revolting sound-effects, this cough was very definitely productive.

'Ooo 'ou 'an 'o oo' a' i?' said Joe, holding on to wherever was unlucky enough to be in his mouth, a residence even a gob of sputum might find uncongenial. I interpreted this as 'Do you want to look at it?'

I considered this. On the one hand, patient satisfaction; Joe clearly needed his suffering witnessed and validated (if you cough up green phlegm in the forest, and there is no-one there to hear it, who gives a damn?). On the other hand, my own mental health could be at risk.

'It would be the highlight of my life, Joe,' I said eventually, on the rationale that (a) I try to be A Good Doctor, and (b) after the spectacle of Joe expectorating noisily into a little jar, the day couldn't get any worse.

We looked at the final result. In silence. It sat on the desk and looked back at us. It was disappointing; clear as a mountain stream it was.

Joe was devastated, he'd obviously been hoping for something leprechaun green, green as the meadows of Alt-na-Brocaigh after the farmers have dumped fertiliser upstream, which would have qualified him for an antibiotic.

'It's pretty clear, Joe,' I confirmed. 'So clear that Cleopatra could have taken a bath in it before hooking up with Mark Anthony.'

'Would you like me to have another go?' said Joe gamely, beginning to hawk violently again. As Samuel Beckett might have said, 'Gob. Fail. Gob again. Fail better.' Honestly, if Tony Blair had had Joe's backbone, he would have refused to be Bush's pet, and the Iraq invasion and the consequent mess might never have happened.

'It must be only a virus, ain't that great?' I said, rubbing it in.

As Sun Tzu said in *The Art of War*: 'Never give the enemy a second chance.'

Looking after (my own) mental health…

GP 31 October 2007

'I'm here about my mental health,' said Joe.

'No, seriously,' I said.

'Seriously,' he said, 'I'm here about my mental health.'

There was a long silence (I'm good at these, I usually close my eyes, maybe grab a quick nap) while I waited for elaboration.

Eventually; 'There was an ad on TV last night, all these people saying how important your mental health was and how you had to look after it, and then at the end it said you were to go and see your doctor, and all.'

Another long silence.

Eventually; 'So what are you going to do about it?' he asked.

My screen is deliberately out of the eye-line of my patients, because lay people wouldn't understand the complicated information (such as Med3 x 4/52, LBP; you need years of study and heaps of letters after your name to understand that).

And it would distract them. I want my patients to be free to concentrate fully on my non-verbal cues; folded arms, impatient tapping of feet, irritated glances at the clock, yawns, and vast and almost elephantine borborygmi. As the world grows smaller, universal body language has assumed greater importance.

So, comfortably out of sight, I googled 'mental health'.

'Try and find the courage to change the things you can and the serenity to accept the things you can't, and the wisdom to know the difference,' I began.

He seemed impressed, my TV experience of reading an autocue while making it seem like spontaneous and inane chatter came in handy.

I was getting into my stride now.

'Yea, though you walk through the valley of the shadow of death, on second thoughts, don't walk, run, as you get through the valley quicker that way; and the lion shall lay down with the lamb, though only the lion will get up the next morning; and now is the winter of your discontent made summer by the glorious ... glorious good weather we've been having lately; and always look on the bright side, life is like a box of chocolates, you never know what you're going to get next; and you can't always get what you want, uh-huh, uh-huh, but if you try sometimes, you get what you need.'

'Thanks doc,' he said, getting up, an enlightened look on his face, as if he just visited the biggest buddha in the world, 'You've certainly given me a lot to think about.'

'Live long and prosper, Spock,' I said.

Chapter 6

The science of relaxation

Just as there is more to patients than simply being patients, there is more to doctors than simply being doctors. There are times when we throw off the iron chains of duty and are more like real people....

The session

BMJ 20 December 1997

One of the joys of Irish culture is our music sessions. You stagger out of the lashing rain into a pub, someone is playing in the corner; you grab a beer, whip out your harpoon or your guitar and get involved. More fun than Disneyland, more team spirit than the SAS, particularly at our annual folk festival, where we have never had any problems with the paramilitaries. 'We know where you live,' we threaten them, 'and we'll come and play outside your house.'

There is a downside; music is in our blood, they say, but so is cholesterol, and years of clandestine observation has led to the conclusion that there are many hidden dangers involved, and every instrument has its own unique hazards. The Corner House in Rostrevor has provided me with the following observational data, and any resemblance to persons alive or dead is right on the money.

Guitar—A gentleman has been defined as someone who doesn't play his guitar at a session. It is a perilous diversion; if you play it badly the other musicians will hate you; if you play it well the other guitarists—that is, 90%

of the other musicians—will hate you. So beware of being mugged on the way home. Bring bandages and antiseptic, and get insured.

Uileann pipes—For some bizarre, unfathomable reason beautiful, exotic foreign women find grotesquely sweaty, hairy, ruddy featured men, maniacally pumping their right elbow, irresistibly attractive. So before rushing out for lessons, stop at the chemist for supplies.

Fiddle—Virtuosos, believing that all others are there only to give them backing, can develop paranoid delusions of supremacy and rush out at any moment to receive imaginary awards. May need sedation. Their 'flying right elbow' can cause eye, skull, and dental injuries to unwary neighbours.

Double bass—He-men, they moonlight as lumberjacks and have wrists thicker than a fiddler's waist, which they could wrench as easily as a chicken's neck. Luckily, they are gentle and easily intimidated. Can get splinters, so bring tweezers and local anaesthetic.

Bodhran—A kind of drum. The instrument of last resort, for those who can play nothing else, and basically an excuse to hang out with the band and drink. These unfortunate individuals are prone to depression, because everyone else, even the guitarists, at worst despises and at best feels pity towards them—that is, 'pity we've no shotgun.' Bullet proof clothing is advisable, and be ready to borrow the bass man's tweezers to extract the pellets from your arse.

Accordion—The musical equivalent of an infectious, purulent skin rash, which is a bizarre coincidence as they sweat profusely with the effort required to carry the damn thing and are prone to develop infectious, purulent skin rashes.

Banjo—Suffer from a chronic inferiority complex, but, as they constantly reassure themselves, at least they ain't guitarists. Hate mandolin players for associated reasons. Are shy with girls and drink too much, so not an advisable instrument for single men with addictive personalities. Usually have domineering mothers and make particularly pathetic and offensively melancholic drunks.

Tin whistle—Prone to falling forward when stuporous and consequently liable to teeth and palate injury, as the whistle is usually still in position. Gumshields are advised and, uniquely, may improve their appearance.

Flute—Slobber a lot, so other musicians must sit some distance away lest body fluids are inadvertently exchanged. It is stating the obvious that they are usually farmers.

Mandolin—Bags of street cred, but as this instrument is utterly inaudible, the musician often wears a wet T shirt to attract attention. Chronic chest problems are a consequence.

It is indeed a perverse and bizarre world where you need a licence to own a dog, yet any fool can play a bodhran. But are we simply avoiding intimacy issues in a fog of wild ceilidh tunes and whiskey fumes? And who wants to be there when the music stops? Do I have to say I love you in a song?

Footnote; Dedicated to my buddies in the Corner House; Matthew, Alfie, Jimmy, Mary, Phil, Claire, Tuesday nights are always rock'n'roll.

Breaking bad (musical) news

BMJ 1 September 2001

Breaking bad news is quite all right with me; as La Rochefoucauld said, 'We all have strength enough to bear the troubles of others.' However, I often try to soften the blow with the gift of music: 'Your Auntie Rose is dead,' sung to the tune of 'Happy Birthday'; or the gift of humour: 'You have two months to live, gosh, but that was from last month, and this is February'; or the gift of charades, which is tricky, as medical terms don't lend themselves to mime—once I had to abandon a consultation prematurely, as the patient was in pain and was nowhere near getting 'You have a whopping big pilonidal sinus.'

But Joe was a tough call. We'd be gently caressing a slow air on the mandolin and whistle and then Joe would come busting in with the 12-string guitar, deafening everyone.

We'd tried many schemes. We'd file his strings so that they'd snap. We'd employ women to chat him up, but Joe was no beauty, Ireland is a small country, and we soon ran out of women. We tried fake phone messages that his granny was dead, which strangely worked the first three times. We suggested he try another instrument, which only led to the Great Accordion Disaster of 1998.

So the band decided Joe would have to be terminated. The band was being compromised, music and beauty were the real losers, and due to my medical training, I was selected to break the bad news.

Sticking my finger down my throat in the graceful Irish gesture of farewell, I left to do the terrible deed.

'Me and the boys were thinking,' I started, 'that maybe you should ...' But the words wouldn't come out. Joe's dog-like face was inches from mine, and I could see a mute appeal in his eyes. Had his senses, so useless when it came to anything musical, subliminally warned him that the knives were out? It felt like kicking a spaniel, of which I have had some experience; the sagging skin under his eyes, the hairs growing out of his ears, the greying of his stubble, Joe was growing old and maybe beneath the bravado lay the fear of not belonging. Perhaps it was fear that made him play so loudly, just as primitive tribes bang drums to frighten away the demons of the night: deep down Joe was afraid that he was no good.

'Joe,' I tried again, 'maybe you should ...' and then I heard myself damn us to a dread musical Götterdämmerung, 'maybe you should bring in the Accordion next week.'

The hippocratic oath, or the honour of the parish?

GP 7 May 2008

The chains of our ancient office lie heavy upon us, but in return for carrying this heavy and eternal burden we receive the respect and esteem of society, and this esteem can be harnessed in many different ways.

Gaelic football is our passion, and last week I attended a game against a neighbouring parish. A few minutes into the match, one of the opposing players became short of breath. I was pointed out to the opposing mentors and they called me over.

It was a very mild asthmatic episode. I had a medical kit with me, for our own team, so after a few theatrical interventions with an inhaler I announced a cure and returned him to the bosom of his team.

The referee thanked me, their coach was grateful, and their chairman came over to shake my hand, saying that this was wonderful example of the GAA community working together, and how it went far beyond mere parish loyalty.

161

Indeed.

In the dying minutes of what was a very close match, an opposition shot whizzed just past the post. Being a (relatively) unimportant match, and consequently there being no goal-net in situ, an uproar ensued.

'Goal,' screamed the opposition.

'Wide,' howled the home supporters.

The referee was some distance up the field and it was an impossible call for him. He needed an objective opinion from someone who could be trusted, someone would be unbiased, a pillar of the community who wouldn't tell a lie. And in an incredibly lucky break for him, who should be standing right beside the goal-post but the Doctor, whose integrity was beyond dispute and whose bona fides had already been established.

'Wide,' I signalled, 'It was a mile wide.'

Women; after only one thing

GP 20 May 2015

As La Rochefoucauld said, 'To refuse praise is to wish to be praised twice,' so I was both charmed and delighted to be named *Best Writer in the World Eve*r or something like that at the Periodical Publishers Awards, the Oscars of the magazine world in some big fancy place in London, chandeliers and toadies everywhere.

We salt-of-the-earth family doctors are hard to impress, but it was a very glamorous occasion. The audience were all marketing and media people (and therefore even more glib and superficial than me), the women slick and stylish, the young men smooth and sleek, the older men distinguished; it was like being in a room with a thousand drug reps.

As Joanna Lumley read the nominations, each one got a huge cheer from their hordes of supporters; except me, of course, although the lady sitting next to me did give a rather half-hearted 'Wheee!'

Anyway, I won. Pausing only to wave two fingers graciously at the losers, their begrudging applause music to my ears, I crossed the crowded floor to the podium.

It was big room in a big hotel, and by the time I reached the podium Joanna had visibly aged.

'Congratulations,' she said, fondling the lapels of my cheap rented tuxedo, 'Any chance of a few beers after the show?'

'I beg your pardon, madam,' I said, shocked and feeling rather violated, 'I am a doctor, don't you know.'

'Oooooh,' she said clearly impressed, 'A doctor as well as an incredibly brilliant award-winning writer; and so handsome, I just adore the way the theatre lights glisten on your sweaty bald head.'

I grabbed the microphone.

'Thank you, you're a wonderful audience, all those doubted me can kiss my ass....'

'The exit's thataway,' said Joanna, a real pro, trying to wrestle the mike from me. I didn't hear her though (I was too busy being adored) and it was my hour, one far fierce hour and sweet, and I wrestled back. We wrestled away while the audience whooped and hooted and threw coins. We wrestled across the stage, we wrestled out through the back door and into the garden.

Under the stars, the little fire-folk sitting in the sky, her perfume was intoxicating, her beauty elfin and dreamlike. She blew softly in my ear and murmured in a low, husky, thrilling voice; 'I've an awful sore throat; can I have an antibiotic?'

In praise of cows

BMJ 27 January 2010

I don't like hunting, because it's not very sporting; take the guns away from the rednecks, I say. If Sarah Palin strapped on a pair of horns and went head to head with a moose, that would be quite all right with me.

But strap on a pair and take aim at a cow, and the cow will just look on you pityingly. Cows mustn't be very bright. It's obvious, they don't have even have any religion. They are too primitive to understand that there is some big guy up in the sky who made everything and then chucked in a few arbitrary rules about eating fish on Fridays and stoning homosexuals as abominations. But neither do cows ever hurry; they travel at their own pace with aldermanic dignity; they don't have important appointments; they lack the ambition to join the million dollar club and buy that condo in Portugal.

Being delayed by cows is a part of of country life, so when I came up behind Joe magisterially guiding his herd along a narrow road I knew there was no point in getting stressed. Equanimity (or apathy) is one of my chief virtues, along with sarcasm and lust. Like Martin Luther, there I sat; I could do no other but take a few moments out from life's cares, peace dropping slow all about me, lulled by Joe's soft encouraging croon and the gentle sussuration and whish of cow-tails.

Then, for a bit of divilment, I tooted the horn. I saw Joe momentarily stiffen at this unmannerly breach of the country code, then pretend to ignore it, so I tooted again, leant out the window, and shouted, 'Shift those bloody cows out of the way.'

This was too great a provocation; Joe turned and approached the car, his face like thunder.

At the last moment I jumped out. 'Joe,' I said, 'It's me!'

'By the hokey,' said Joe, 'Is it yourself, doctor?'

'It's me, bitch,' I confirmed in my best gangsta rapper jive, and then, in the style of the Pink Panther: ''Ave you a licence for zeeze cows?'

Joe began to laugh, a great unstoppable infectious laugh, and I couldn't help but join in. And as we rolled about in the middle of the road, the cows milled around us, bemused, but happy that we were happy.

And in no hurry to get anywhere.

We cannot defeat our enemies, but we will meet them in battle nonetheless...

GP 26 February 2009

Morning surgeries are always a battle, and each day, as I gird my loins and oil my mighty thews (I usually do this myself, unless there's a complementary therapist about) I think back to my illustrious companions-in-arms Hector and Paris, returning to the plains of windy Troy after a brief and well-deserved dalliance with Helen and Andromache.

Homer, a writer like myself, and therefore prone to slight exaggeration, described it as follows; as a stallion breaks loose and gallops gloriously over the plain, his mane streaming, exulting in his strength, flying like the wind to the haunts of his mares - so forth went Paris from high

Pergamus, and he laughed as he sped swiftly on his way, pausing only to nip back for his prescription pad.

The past has rended us, and we all have our scars, but a scar is not always a flaw. Kintsugi is the Japanese art of repairing broken pottery with lacquer dusted or mixed with powdered gold, so that the apparently shattered object becomes more beautiful than before. A scar may be redemption inscribed in flesh, a memorial to something endured, something forever lost but something intangible gained, maybe a layer of invisible armour.

I've suffered many defeats and humiliations, but I'm still here, my armour accreted over the long bitter years, so the slings and arrows of outrageous fortune don't bother me, and this equanimity is a virtue for GPs, as no human concern is so trivial and bizarre that it can't be dumped on us.

But even Homer nods, and I was idly musing about GP heaven (interesting cases, grateful patients, no out of hours, long coffee breaks, jam doughnuts) when Mrs O'Toole came in. My defences were momentarily down, and like any predator, she could sense vulnerability.

'It's the hole in the ozone layer; in the Arctic, you know,' she began.

I sighed: 'Thinking of moving there?'

'I'm very worried about it,' she persisted.

'This is Ireland,' I said. 'It'll just mean more rain.'

'And then there's global warming, and flooding,' she continued, undaunted.

'You live halfway up a mountain,' I reminded her, my clinical instincts briefly resurfacing; reassurance is a therapeutic modality and sometimes it's all we've got.

'And oil, what'll we do when the oil runs out and all?'

'The Arctic's supposed to be really nice,' I suggested.

F(r)iends

BMJ 16 December 1995

One of the great joys, and at the same time one of the great sorrows, of a medical career is the many friends we make and the many friends we lose. The nature of the job forges the deepest bonds; young people stressed to their breaking point, sharing long hours, warm bodies, and late nights, we get to know each other as we truly are. Our hopes and dreams, our fears and insecurities--sharing them came as naturally as surviving. A war situation was no place for reticence or foreplay, and, despised by everyone else, we had to stick together to endure.

And then, the nature of the job meant we would move on after six months. For a while we would stay in touch, maybe meet sometimes for a few beers and to rake over old times, nostalgia softening the memories of exhaustion and humiliation; then the pressures of time and distance would become too strong, and the new friendships we were building in our new trenches would take their place.

I had one particular group of friends in college; we had a poker school every week and we diligently skipped lectures to attend racecourses all over Ireland. Fairyhouse, Punchestown, Kilbeggan - the names still roll like music off my tongue and conjure a little tear in my eye, redolent with the scent of cheap whiskey and cigars, and the silky texture of torn bookies' dockets. Ah, that unforgettable day when Patsy's potential jackpot winner fell at the final fence; the expression on his face was like one of those Greek plays where everybody dies, his acceptance of our profuse commiserations rather less than gracious. As La

Rochefoucauld observed, 'There is in the misfortune of one's friends something not entirely unpleasant.'

But through all these good times we somehow believed that the best was yet to come; when we qualified, and had some spending money, we'd be able to do whatever we wanted; Cheltenham, Saratoga, Longchamp--what fun, what excitement we would have. But it hasn't worked out that way; first our jobs, now our families have separated us. We have been displaced to exotic destinations all over the world--Saskatoon, Perth, Boston, Crossmaglen; and I don't think we'll ever all get together again.

When we are young it seems that we can do anything we want; we have freedom but no funds, dreams but no resources. But as we get older and our authority grows so do our responsibilities, and our options become more and more limited. Until it comes to the point where our duties allow us no choices anymore; we have children to support, patients to look after, absolute obligations we must fulfil.

So at the last there is only that one thing which we must do, that one course which we must follow--and it ain't a racecourse.

How do you want to be remembered?

BMJ 22 November 1997

How strong you were, so bright and gay / A prince of love in every way / Ah yes—I remember it well. — Gigi

Africa: the name alone inspires and magicks, a land redolent of spice and wild beasts, where champions stalked and men of rock like Burton and Stanley roamed. And it has its very own guardian angel: high in the plateau above Ngorongoro Crater is a simple stone monument to Michael Grzimek.

With his father, Bernard, he was among the first to recognise the precious jewel that the east African reserves represent and the mortal danger they were in; together father and son fought tirelessly to save them and to inform an unsuspecting and apathetic world of the impending crisis.

But those whom the gods love die young; if you listen hard enough you can hear the angel's wings, and Michael Grzimek was killed tragically at the age of 28, when his small aircraft crashed on the Serengeti Plains, perhaps after a collision with a vulture. His portrait hangs in the lodge overlooking Ngorongoro Crater, 9000 feet high in the Rift Valley escarpment; a boyish smile, teeth gleaming, eyes bright, flying scarf streaming out in the wind, his youthfulness enshrined, captured forever, age never to wither him, a young Adonis in the fields of the Lord.

A book that strongly influenced me was Blake Morrison's And When Did You Last See Your Father? Evocative, disturbing in his brutal honesty, Morrison talks about his father's death from cancer, and of the last time he saw him as he really was, before illness overtook him. His father, a GP, was a big, burly, practical man, and Morrison last remembers him hanging a chandelier and then saying, 'Excellent. What's the next job then?'

It's a message I try to pass on to my own patients. I'm always disturbed by the two kinds of corpse we see in the coffin after a long neoplastic illness; they either seem to be cachectic and wasted or fat and bloated by steroids, but in either case almost unrecognisable and not representative of the person they once were.

So when their father or mother or sister or friend is lying in the coffin I take them aside and say to them, 'Don't remember him that way, not the way he looks now—he wouldn't want that—and don't remember him either as a sick man, and don't use a recent photo of him for the memorial cards, his face creased, a strained smile, his clothes looking two sizes too big for him. Use an old photo for the cards; remember him as he used to be, healthy, ruddy faced, vigorous, leaping over a ditch in the country, holding up his children, laughing in a crowd at a wedding—think about him the way you want to— think of him the way he truly was. Death is just a coda at the end of the life, it doesn't make that life any less worth the living.'

***

And when I saw Michael Grzimek's picture I thought, 'That's how I'd like to be remembered.'

And then I thought, 'Yea, I could murder a Big Mac.'

Colonoscopy (1); damned uncomfortable

GP 16 April 2009

Do you remember the good old days, when men were men and GI investigations meant something? When you only organised a colonoscopy or barium enema when you were pretty sure that something would show up. When these procedures demanded drinking four litres of slop the night before. Patients were appreciative of this; anything so unpleasant and disgusting just had to be good for you.

I remember as a student in Dublin being at a demonstration of the first colonoscopy in Ireland. Some social-climbing surgeon had been to America for few weeks and had come back, not only with a Yankee accent, but with a new-fangled way of things.

It was a massive occasion; the patient/victim (how did they get consent for that one?) had had their bowel religiously purged, and the gallery was packed with eager yet sceptical faces.

The scepticism grew to epidemic proportions when we saw the size of the implement. There was a gasp of horror when the surgeon pulled out a thing as big as your fist, which wouldn't have been out of place in a slasher movie. Someone fainted at the back and was enjoyably trampled.

The theatre nurses wheeled the patient in and turned him on his side, his anus blossoming like a dark rose before us, utterly unaware of the honour being bestowed upon it.

The surgeon began inserting the scope, all the while explaining how simple and pain-free the procedure was. Unfortunately, it quickly became clear that the patient was insufficiently anaesthetised.

'It hurts,' whimpered the victim, writhing and wriggling in a doomed attempt to escape his date with destiny, which in the real world might have been reckoned a criminal assault.

'No, it doesn't, you're fine, you're doing great, you can hardly feel a thing.' The surgeon ignored his pleas, taking the opportunity to shove the scope another few centimetres up the arse. The whimpers turned to agonised screams, an almost musical counterpoint to the sniggers of the medical students.

'Stop! Please stop!' begged the patient. 'You're fine, you're fine,' insisted the surgeon, and the dance continued until someone took pity on the victim and set off the fire alarm.

And as the crowd rushed to the exit, 'That's the face of the future,' the surgeon announced grandly.

Colonoscopy (2); the bright side

BMJ   23 September 2000

We doctors are human and frail, so we understand human frailty. In the same way we can truly comprehend illness only when we have been ill ourselves; intellectual knowledge is no substitute for bitter experience.

A few years ago, I had a colonoscopy. The procedure itself was no problem and even the anal catharsis was passable, almost a pleasant diversion, like a walk in the country (albeit the country of the very weird). Thomas More, in his *Utopia*, described defaecation as being one of the primary physical pleasures, though I reckon such an extreme expression of this activity was not quite what he had in mind.

However, despite these pleasant memories, drinking three litres of laxative the night before is an ordeal every doctor should himself endure before inflicting it on others. The advice leaflet recommends that the solution be chilled, but trust me, ice cold glop tastes just as bad as lukewarm glop.

And a further Bright Side; the gastroenterologist generously sent me some lovely pictures of my colon. Call me Narcissus, but the portfolio is as soft focused as a South Sea sunset; romantic, roseate, like a Martian cavern with disco lights, a hint of mystery behind every nook and crevice, the kind of place you could come around a corner and suddenly encounter Humphrey Bogart and Peter Lorre engaged in furtive conversation.

Not that there are any crevices, for the mucosal surface is as slick and smooth as a New Labour spin doctor; the walls not too mucusy, not too dry. If my colon were a footballer, Barcelona and Juventus would be begging for my signature. I'd be a superstar, perhaps release an auto-biography, write a best-selling novel (if Jeffrey Archer can do it, why not my colon?), then the tabloids would be on my trail, perhaps exposing an illicit lavage, some compromising pictures of my colon in bed with Liz Hurley, then I'd be ruined; perhaps I'm taking this analogy too far.

So attractive though the pictures were, I don't boast about them, nor show them off to my friends; there are some things a man just has to keep to himself, parts of the body too private and personal for public display, parts of the body even the most enthusiastic and uninhibited nudist would feel uncomfortable about advertising.

My colon and I must remain undiscovered.

Happiness

British Journal of General Practice, October 2000

Now that I don't travel by Concorde anymore, my second career as a media superstar requires a lot of driving, and I have found that nothing shortens the journey like a good audio-book. Get involved and the time flies, you'll nearly be sorry you've arrived. My tastes are eclectic, from Dickens to *The X-Files*, from Anthony Trollope to Michael Crichton, but most of all I recommend the slow mid-western drawl of Garrison Keillor.

His essays about the mythical town of Lake Wobegone in Minnesota are at the same time soothing and stimulating, comic and philosophic. Lake Wobegone, he tells us, was settled over a hundred years ago by a group of immigrant Norwegian farmers, and their descendants are, as Keillor observes with the occasional, reluctant trace of affection, a dour people of very few words.

I can sympathise; during my years of general practice I have come to share some of these Norwegian virtues, as I am increasingly suspicious of people who are too happy-go-lucky (I'm not happy, I'm not lucky, and I don't go). They either know something I don't or they are repressing and ready to explode.

A patient of mine is a folk-singer, and accordingly manifests both the irritating tweeness and the indefatigable optimism demanded by the accursed breed. I reckon it's mainly due to all those years of being dandled on his granny's knee; at forty-two he's a bit old to be still at it, but the old lady remains hale and hearty and by now has thigh muscles so well developed they could crack walnuts.

Nothing seems to get him down and his cheerfulness is almost pathological. Lashing rain is a 'soft day, thank God'; something bad happening merits, 'If that's the worst thing that happens to us today, we've had a good day'; something *really* bad happening earns, 'At least I'm not Scottish.'

I imagine telling him some day, 'Tadhg, I have some bad news for you. It's about your dog, the one you sat up all night delivering and who has been your inseparable companion and only consolation since your wife passed away so tragically all those years ago and who only last week saved your father from being asphyxiated by a rancid peccary; I regret to say I've just run her down and she is far beyond resuscitation on account of you normally needing your head not being squashed for that to work.'

He'd be silent for a while, maybe a little sob for theatrical purposes, then look up at me with a twinkle in his eyes (you can't learn that twinkle, and surgical attempts to recreate it have only ended up with an evil squint) and a plucky smile and say, 'You know, Doc, when I was just a wee lad my grand-daddy used to sing a song about that while he was teaching me how to scratch my eyeballs with a fork', and he'd close his eyes, switching off the twinkle for a moment, and start to croon in a voice that was full of anguish, pain, and sorrow but yet strangely also full of joy and wonder and sodomy (his emotions were a little mixed up, you may gather) and a hope for a new tomorrow that maybe would also bring a new dog:

'The driver ran over my dog', he'd lilt, 'It was the driver's door that caught her/But every cloud has a silver lining/He reversed over Harry Potter/Toor-aloor-a-loora, jiggety-jiggetty-jig.'

Simultaneously laughing and crying he'd hug me close to his suspiciously quivering bosom, and whisper, 'By the way, I have to kill you now,' the sun glinting merrily on the carving knife.

'Mirth is always good and cannot be excessive', said Spinoza, but as Garrison Keillor's Norwegian farmers might retort, what would he know about it?

Doctor in Tights

GP 9 July 2009

I belong to an amateur drama society; though I am good at remembering lines and am therefore dependable, I am also as wooden as Pinocchio and incapable of conveying any emotion (except for apathy, of course, I've had years of practice at that). For this reason, and also because of my inborn aldermanic dignity and because I am good at shouting, I usually get minor authority roles, such as the judge or the lord of the manor.

One medieval drama required me to wear tights. I'm cool with that, but on the first night there was a reception beforehand. When we GPs get involved with anything we are inevitably voted in as chairperson (folks seem to think it's a big deal that we belong to an ancient and noble profession, revered for its wisdom and scholarship) I was required to mingle. This left me little time to change for the performance, so to save a few minutes, I wore my tights underneath my trousers.

And it was an epiphany; the almost imperceptible sussuration of tights against trousers was unexpectedly sensual. I felt like a cross between Fred Astaire and Cyd Charisse, more aware of my own body, the beguiling curves, the rippling muscles, my walk became a strut, my movements panther-like. The tights had the curious effect of seeming to firm up my buttocks, giving them more definition, making them look harder, more toned. It also seemed to have a significant effect on the ladies present; I caught quite a few sideways glances, unashamedly checking me out, as if they liked the cut of my jib.

'Have you been working out?' asked one.

'Nice buns,' said another.

I looked good, I felt dangerous, lean and hungry as Cassius, the fatal glamour of the stage the ultimate aphrodisiac.

So, lads, try on the tights at least once before you die, and as physicians we must also remember their value as a therapeutic tool. Any man who comes in complaining of low mood and low self-esteem (let's face it, we all suffer from this, it's only real losers and mammy's boys who have to go running to the doctor whining about it), don't reach for the prescription pad or the referral letter, don't bore them with banal lectures about lifestyle, just advise them to slip on a pair of tights.

Maybe try it at home first.

Footnote; The 'amateur drama society,' was in fact the Rostrevor Cor na Nog, run by my sister Siubhan, who is a musical genius and should really be in Hollywood, and her great friend and sparring partner Eibhlis Mills. This particular event was in Malta, but they've also performed in Monte Carlo and Madrid, where, strangely, they kept me backstage.

The Skelligs (1); if you have one day in Ireland...

GP   July 21 2012

'If you do one thing in Ireland, visit the Skellig Islands,' said the boatman, Thomas Bawn Brosnan, sea-weathered and ruddy-faced and unruffled by the choppy seas.

Ten miles off the Atlantic coast of Ireland, two craggy mountainous islands reared out of the ocean, jagged peaks seeming to claw at the sky. White sea-birds wheeled along the cliffs, buffeted by the freshening breeze. The sky was overcast, the sea the colour of iron. Dwarfed by the elements, our boat slipped past the smaller island, Skellig Beag, a maelstrom of glimmering wings, home to thousands of gannets; the bobbing heads of seals were everywhere and the sea was alive with rafts of puffins and shearwaters. The cries of the sea-birds were almost deafening, counterpointed by the sound of the less hardy travellers chucking spectacularly and colourfully over the side (learning point: herring gulls eat vomit).

I climbed the 670 steps along a sheer cliff which led from the small pier to the beehive huts. Fatalities aren't unknown, both from falling over the edge and from the unexpected physical demands of the climb; they should really consider an escalator, even if it is a UNESCO World Heritage Site.

The steps led up to a small gathering of stone beehive huts in which the monks had endured over 600 years of unbelievable hardship, from the sixth century on. I tried to imagine what it would have been like. Vegetation was sparse, tenacious grass and heather only. Autumn would be fierce here, winter a terror. Storms howling in from the Atlantic, bitter cold, driving rain, precious little except birds' eggs and fish and whatever few vegetables they were able to grow, no TV and Sky Sports.

Because of the unsettled weather, there were few visitors. I wandered away from the huts and found myself alone. In the lee of frowning cliffs an apologetic Irish rain drifted down. Choughs flitted bat-like from ledge to ledge. To the east lay Skellig Beag, blushed white with the debris of countless nests; to the west lay only the trackless ocean. I closed my eyes, listening; Skellig Michael had its own ancient voice, the crashing waves, the sea-birds' cries, the capricious breeze dancing among the cliffs and whistling among the rocks.

I crossed a grassy slope swarming with puffins, their burrows thick all around me. A large puffin chick peeped out of a burrow. Its parent flew in, and responded to the begging behaviour in textbook fashion by regurgitating slops. The chick got most of it, but some spilled on the ground.

A greater black-backed gull swooped down to gobble up the spill. Greater black-backed gulls steal food from smaller and less aggressive creatures, such as kittiwakes, puffins and dwarves. But the gull went a step further; it grabbed the chick by its leg and started to drag it from the burrow. The chick squealed, the parent fluttered in alarm, but they were over-matched.

I was in a quandary; if this was a wildlife documentary, I'd be conscientious, agonising that the brutal scene was all part of the natural world. Interfering would be academically incorrect. The gull also had to eat and probably had chicks of its own. But viewing nature through this prism is becoming less and less realistic; humans interfere in everything and nature has to adapt to our presence.

We have entered a new dynamic; gulls have prospered by scavenging our rubbish and devouring our vomit, and puffins may have achieved their own evolutionary edge by being cute and spunky and photogenic. And I'm Irish and we hate bullies, having been bullied by the English for centuries; the Great Hunger was all England's fault, though it was a long time ago and I've kinda gotten over it by now.

I strode over. 'Get away from her, you bitch,' I said, like Ripley in *Aliens*. Not trying to brag, but that gull was one big and scary bird. It reluctantly released the chick's leg and flew away with a resentful squawk. The chick retreated into the burrow, and the parent regarded me with bright eyes for a long and curiously intimate moment. A flock of its comrades whirred above, expectorating over my runners.

That's gratitude for you, I thought.

The Skelligs (2); the most precious gift

BMJ 15 February 1997

A few summers ago a good friend and I took an overnight trip to the Skellig Islands, off the coast of Kerry. We had two reasons. Firstly, we wanted to see the huge puffin and gannet colonies, as we are both children of nature. Secondly, as we are both weird dudes and wanted to get in touch with ourselves, where better to do that than in an eighth century monastery on an island on the edge of the world, in the uttermost west, with nothing between us and America but thousands upon thousands of miles of restless ocean.

On the boat trip out his little daughter came with us. She is badly handicapped due to cerebral palsy. She cannot see or talk, but apart from that has no limitations, and she was the star of the show, standing bolt upright, straight and steadfast as a tree, defying the capriciously lurching ship, her balance perfect, her smile as bright as a sun burst.

'She enjoys the feel of the engines throbbing up through the deck, and the sun and breeze and spray on her face,' said my friend.

'How do you know?' I asked.

'I just do,' he said, 'I just know it.'

Later that night, sitting by the camp fire in the shelter of the ruined walls, with the cries of the seabirds, the song of the wind, the storm-tossed half moon above us, I remembered that expression, and our conversation strayed away from women and horse racing and towards that most perilous of all subjects - the truth.

I asked him where he found the strength to bear this cross; to see this beautiful child, his child, so curtailed and restricted. I was consciously revealing my own inner demons here; it is something I have always been uncomfortable with. When faced with a handicapped child I feel inadequate, helpless, and I move on as soon as I can to something more concrete that I can actually do something about.

'Too busy,' I tell myself, 'So much to do; so little time.' But I do not leave the guilt behind so easily; I carry it with me. So how could he bear such a thing, hour after hour, day after day, year after year, with no chance of ever seeing any improvement in her condition?

'She gives me this great gift,' he answered. 'Every day I pick her up, I hug her, I tickle her, and I hear her laughter, like the peal of bells on a frosty morning; and hour after hour, day after day, year after year, I will do these things; for this is the gift she gives me, beyond any price, worth any burden.

'Without guile, without reserve, she allows me to love her.'

Footnote; dedicated to my late friend Michael Corry.

Much doth it profit a subtle doc

BMJ 10 May 2003

My native village of Rostrevor dates to pre-Christian times, and the Farrell clan have been here all along, a savage race as ancient and atavistic as the peat; to us the good old days means hunter-gathering, not poncing about in fake Victorian costumes. The ancestral Farrells used to own all the land, until it was stolen from us by the Druids.

Gaelic football is our passion; my son Jack now wears the same red and black worn by his father and his father's father before him, and I am one of the team mentors. Mentor was Telemachus' adviser during Ulysses' suspiciously protracted return from Troy, and I am sure that if deep-browed Homer could have foreseen how Mentor's name would be hijacked by a bunch of overweight balding men running up and down the touchline in unflattering pink lycra, he would have been both charmed and delighted.

The role of team doctor is a broad church. Of course, I treat injuries and advise on fitness etc, but when the honour of the parish is at stake, the Hippocratic oath becomes but a trifling matter.

Last year we reached the county final, and on the big day I introduced myself beforehand to the referee, assuring him that my medical skills were available to both sides if needed, thus winning him with honest trifles to betrayals of deeper consequence. It proved a wise investment.

Rostrevor was two points ahead with only minutes left, when one of the Twin Magees (I still can't tell them apart) went down from an accidental boot to the ear. In emergency medicine every second counts, and I burst on to the field to gasps from the crowd.

Sprinting desperately, I arrived just in time before the brat got up, pushing him back down with one heavy hand while putting on a Robert Jones bandage with the other (this was a cunning and time consuming choice).

Aware of the thin line between safely running down the clock and the referee smelling a rat, I timed it carefully. I tied the last knot with a flourish and seconds later the final whistle blew, the other mentors surged forward and carried me shoulder high on a glorious lap of honour, and we drank the blood of our enemies and exulted in the lamentations of their women-folk.

'Let me have around me men that are fat,' I thought.

Footnote; Dedicated to my good friends Tom Magee, Dominic Tinnelly, Paddy McAvoy, Paul McGrath, Peter

Bailey and Brian Fitzpatrick, with whom I have spent many happy years running up and down the line.

When doctors strike back

GP 29 August 2014

We crossed a small but significant Rubicon last week. Physical attacks on doctors have been increasing, the armour of our non-combatant status shedding its potency more and more with each day that passes.

There are times when such attacks might be predictable - a night call down a dark alley, a drink-crazed lager lout in A&E, an overly territorial sheep. But how about this for an unlikely scenario? A football stadium, 50,000 in attendance, millions more watching on TV.

At the All-Ireland GAA football quarter-final, in Croke Park in Dublin, between Donegal and Armagh, the Donegal doctor was sent flying by an Armagh player. The doctor displayed admirable equanimity, picking himself up with what was left of his dignity and refusing to complain either during or after the match.

But was this the right response? Must we always turn the other cheek? I'm a lover, not a fighter, but it's time to make a stand.

If I'd been the doctor, I would have got up slowly, waited until the player's back was turned (he was a big lad), then slugged him from behind, before beating a quick retreat to the safety of the dug-out. As Terry Pratchett observed, 'I wish everyone was brave enough to be as cowardly as me.'

Unprofessional behaviour, I hear you say, but no, this would have been preventive medicine at its finest. Attack a doctor again, it would say, and see what you get, when your back is turned, you are doomed - dark things come out at night and your lifelong terror will be perfectly reasonable.

We'd explain our actions, of course; keeping patients informed is a cornerstone of the doctor/patient relationship. And it won't hurt too much, we're using a blunt needle, see? We would never condone violence in any form.

Except when we do it, naturally.

Make Comets Great Again

BMJ 11 September 1999

Those were the days: the Apollo missions, fuzzy pictures from the moon, *Also Sprach Zarathustra*, James Burke, and Patrick Moore jumping up and down with an ingenuous and guileless excitement that was irresistibly infectious. It seemed that a new age was dawning, and the uncluttered truths of science would provide all the answers.

But the blissful unimpeached Arcady was not to last, and because of this the word 'comet' to me has never suggested a magnificent ball of fire hurtling across the solar system, with a shimmering silver tail a million miles long. Rather it implies shattered dreams and busted expectations, because I remember all too clearly the bitter disappointment of Comet Kohoutek in the 1970s (and also, a sheer coincidence, that no girls would go out with me).

'It'll be half the size of the moon,' enthused Patrick Moore, who had never lied to me before, and whom I—still just a kid with stars in my eyes—really believed. But my faith in him and my boyhood dreams were to be utterly betrayed, for when Comet Kohoutek eventually arrived it was as ineffectual as a cough bottle from the *British National Formulary*.

And the busted expectations continued: antibiotics, interferon, Ben Johnson; morning glories with feet of clay.

So I had no hopes for Comet Hale-Bopp whatsoever, despite all the advance publicity. I'd heard that song before, and it had broken my youthful heart, so I didn't even bother looking up in the sky for it. Until one night, I was lamenting my disenchantment over a few beers with my good friend Petie.

'You mean you haven't seen it yet?' he said in surprise. 'It's been up there for two months now.'

'Well, where is it then?' I said, wondering when exactly he had become such an astronomical expert, if he was as busy looking after his cows as he said he was.

'It's right over my house,' he said emphatically.

Very droll for a hillbilly, I thought, but the very next night I was travelling over the mountains and I stopped the car to look, and… there it was, shining like a beacon in the sky, tail streaming out like a little piece of heaven, Comet Hale-Bopp in a rainbow of glory, and, as promised, right above Petie's house.

Dreams do come true, Dorothy, and sometimes right in our own backyard.

Chapter 7

One guy's opinion(s)

Changing your mind is not de rigeur in Ulster, although we are not unique in this regard. You never see a panellist on questions and answers programmes sit back thoughtfully, and say, "Yes, you're right, that's a good point, it hadn't occurred to me. OK, you've convinced me, I'm changing my mind." It takes strength and wisdom to modify fixed views; weakness and prejudice to persist with them.

The Sufis tell of the mythical idiot savant, Nasruddin Khan, who was once asked his age.

"Fifty years old today," he stated proudly.

Ten years later the same person again inquired about his age.

"Fifty years old," said Nasruddin Khan stoutly. "No doubt about it."

"But that's what you told me 10 years ago," said the surprised questioner.

Replied Nasruddin Khan, "I always stand by what I have said."

So I always have more than one opinion, just to be safe.

A Cure for Cancer?

GP 14 March 2014

Two cavemen were sitting by their cooking fire. One of them leaned back, belching with satisfaction.

'Ain't it great?' he said, 'Clean air, a varied diet, water from mountain streams, no pollution, plenty of exercise, talk about a healthy lifestyle, you couldn't beat it with a big stick.'

'Yes,' agreed the other, 'But isn't it strange how we all die before we reach 30?'

Compared to previous generations, we live lives of unprecedented comfort, safety and longevity, and we don't even need to go back to cavemen to appreciate this. At his time, King Philip of Spain was the most powerful man in the world. His empire stretched across the globe and he had an army of vassals waiting on his every whim. Yet his dying was a thing of horror; wasting away with bed-sores on ordure-drenched sheets for 52 days. He could not be washed because of the pain; thus a hole was cut in his mattress for the release of excrement, urine, pus and blood. Today even the meanest of our citizens would not have to endure such a terrible death.

Not that doctors can claim too much credit for these improvements; it's more thanks to scientific advances in other fields. Farmers contributed more food, engineers provided sanitation and clean water. Apart from the occasional war, science has been good to us. Doctors might make a difference in individual cases, but only our public health colleagues can lay claim to any population-wide effect.

The WHO recently published a report about the increased incidence of cancer; a 'tidal wave' they called it, in unnecessarily emotive language, ignoring the obvious fact that cancer rates are increasing mainly because we are living long enough to develop it; and you could say the same for all the modern epidemics, heart disease, stroke, dementia etc.

There's a reason the menopause occurs in late forties; it's a sign that Mother Nature is finished with us, that our bodies are obsolete, that it's time to move over and make way for our children and that living longer places us in a situation our bodies weren't designed to cope with. So I do have one, perhaps controversial, solution to the 'tidal wave' of cancer.

We could stop childhood vaccinations.

The real enemy of writing, sex and medicine...

GP 21 March 2017

According to research (for which I could list the references if required, even if no-one ever bothers to ask, although references are like nice wallpaper, or having Emeritus before your name, they always add a bit of tone, a bit of scientific gravitas, don't you think?), if we reckon on 15 minutes per consultation, a family doctor with 2,500 patients would spend 7.4 hours per day to deliver all recommended preventive care and 10.6 hours per day to deliver all recommended chronic care.

This leaves a generous six hours every day for that pesky acute care, looking after the worried well, sick certs, sick kids, paperwork, eating, sleeping, banging our heads against the wall in sheer frustration, toileting and reproducing.

The truth is, you can get a lot done when you don't have, you know, a life.

And even our six hours of freedom are under threat; no research paper worth its salt can ever finish without the words 'GPs should...'. The 'recommended' care by outside experts with zero understanding of the realities of primary care continues to pile up.

Yet we continue to accept it, like Boxer in *Animal Farm*, we put our shoulders to the plough and resolve to work harder; it's not our nature to complain, to say no.

Come in and put your feet up, we say instead, and bring your recommendation with you, we have a nice spot for it beside the hearth. When you want something done, ask a busy doc.

But it's time to say stop, we can't do this anymore, it's too much. There is a wonderful German word: *verschlimmbessern*, which means 'to make something worse by trying to improve it'. By striving to make general practice ever better, we are making it an impossible task.

'If we want things to stay as they are,' said Tancredi, 'things will have to change.

As in so many things, from writing columns to having sex to being a family doctor, perfect is the enemy of good.

The imbalanced search for balance

BMJ 23 Jun 2010

Northern Ireland's minister for culture once wrote to the Ulster Museum urging it to reflect creationist and intelligent design theories of the universe's origins. While being interviewed about this on BBC radio he was ambushed by Richard Dawkins, whose withering scorn reduced the minister to an incoherent babbling about intolerance and equality and the need for debate. It was funny but also embarrassing; yep, that's our minister for culture, folks, don't it make you proud?

It also illustrates the dangers of a politically correct search for balance. When the director of the CERN Institute is interviewed about the hadron collider and the nature of the universe, you don't expect an alternative view from Mrs Poots from Barking, who believes that quarks are little white mice that can scurry very fast and that the hadron collider obviously wasn't going to work because the scientists didn't put out enough cheese. The interviewer then turns to the director.

'So, why didn't you put out enough cheese, Mr Scientist?' he asks accusingly.

In science there is no point in debating with nonsense and superstition; even entering a debate lends the nonsense an undeserved credibility. Medicine is particularly susceptible to those who peddle the illusion of knowledge to the gullible and the vulnerable; consider MMR versus anti-MMR, homoeopathy versus medicine that actually works, the tooth fairy versus regular dental hygiene, Santa Claus versus your parents buying stuff, female circumcision, astrology, the stork theory of making babies. It's not even lies, it's just . . . bullshit. At least a lie has some relationship with the truth (being the opposite of it, though operating in the same space), while bullshit is just imaginary nonsense.

Science acknowledges uncertainty, so I'll allow that I might be wrong. Some of these mightn't be just fairy tales; the tooth fairy could be a very hardworking lady; and it's theoretically possible that there's a big fat beardy guy at the North Pole who can warp time and space. If there are so many imitators, as with Elvis, then yes, Virginia, there must be a real Santa Claus somewhere.

There, you see, I'm being properly scientific, always ready to change my mind when presented with credible evidence.

OK, I know this isn't fair, I'm being narrowminded, I've sold out to The Man, I'm under the thumb of Big Pharma; but you'll have to forgive my cynicism, I can't help it.

I'm a Scorpio.

Opera sucks

GP 6 June 2012

When I was a lad and as yet not fully formed, I had musical aspirations, and my big chance came when I sang the part of Momus, the God of Mischief, in Luigi Rossi's *L'Orfeo*. Unfortunately, I was not a success; in those days being ripped and extraordinarily good-looking wasn't enough to compensate for a lack of talent. One critic even had the infernal cheek to say that the God of Mischief sang out of pitch; obviously he didn't understand the art of improvisation, or perhaps I should have used more body oil.

So my operatic career was terminated at an early stage, the silver lining proving to be a big boost to the medical profession, and ever since I've regarded opera as plain stupid. If you need to say something, come right out and say it, no need to burst into song, it's just annoying.

Opera only sounds impressive and exotic because we don't understand the language; 'I'm running to the toilet all day,' sounds pretty dull and mundane, but, using Google Translate, it comes out as *'Sto facendo il bagno tutto il giorno.'* Get some big fat guy with a goatee to sing a few bars of that and the chattering classes will be swooning in the aisles and paying £500 a pop at the door.

Not that our profession is any better; we shamelessly exploit the same device. All professions are conspiracies against the laity, said GB Shaw in The Doctor's Dilemma, and we protect our knowledge with arcane and opaque language designed to mystify and confuse our patients. A heart attack is a myocardial infarct, high BP becomes hypertension, joint pain becomes arthralgia, Marathon becomes Snickers.

And we disguise our ignorance by the same method, for example, chronic muscle pain becomes fibromyalgia. We don't know what causes it, we don't know how to treat it, but we employ a cocktail of Latin and Greek to stick on a fancy name which lends us an illusion of control. It's our very own secret language, and we use it to exclude and disempower mere lay people.

Opera puo succhiare, ma la medicina fa schifo peggio (Opera may suck, but medicine sucks worse).

A poster-boy at last

GP 22 August 2017

The poster presentations at a conference have always seemed rather sad, like the fat kid with glasses who always gets picked last, but keeps turning up nevertheless, doggedly refusing to let the dream die.

The medical version of the sunk cost fallacy, the authors are so emotionally invested in the long thankless hours, the blood, tears and sweat they've committed in the past, they're damned if they're going to give it up.

Not important enough to be allowed on the big stage, but unwilling just to stick their painstaking research in a drawer, they're confined to a little atrium beside the toilets.

Those of us who have been sleeping at the back of the auditorium scurry quickly and heartlessly past as the authors desperately try to catch our eye. It's vital to avoid eye contact at all costs, otherwise someone else will get to the doughnuts first. So during each coffee and lunch break, the poster-boyz are forced to endure this ritual humiliation.

I'm old enough to remember the posters being a whirl of coloured crayons and stencils; now they're the same whirl, but computer-generated, and the posters are still so ultra-congested and dense you could eat them to stay regular.

By far my most memorable poster was 'Effect on the peri-anal mucosa of repeated rectal examinations.' The earnest young man was making it real; he even had a supply of rubber gloves and lubricant, and a fake anal sphincter, which he invited the fascinated yet repulsed spectators to… probe.

There were no takers, so, pity being one of my chief virtues (along with sarcasm and apathy), I stepped forward. I was always taught to be kind to those less fortunate, whether immigrants, refugees or research registrars.

'Feels pretty good to me,' I said, probing deeply.

In accordance with rules of universal humour, someone made a farting noise.

'It can be quite traumatic, you know,' said the poster-boy.

'Interesting,' I told him, in an understatement. 'And your conclusion was that there were no significant changes.'

A lesser man would have been crushed, but this lad was as game as a pebble.

'Oh no,' he said, a gleam in his eye, the gleam of the fanatic which has undermined civilisations and brought great empires crashing down in ruin. 'I'm calling for further research.'

Footnote: Since writing this column, I presented a poster myself, on social media and medicine, at the International Foundation for Integrated Care conference. And yes, I was beside the bathrooms, and yes, everyone ignored me.

Passion required

BMJ 3 April 2008

A few years ago, I felt compelled (out of both a sense of duty and a feeling of nausea) to chide the *Independent* about its complementary health guru.

"Oooh, but he's very popular," was the newspaper's defence.

So is pornography, I said.

"Oooh no," they replied, in an outraged tone, "that wouldn't be ethical," though I reckoned that big tits on page 3 is a lot more ethical than snake oil salesmen peddling the illusion of knowledge to the gullible and the vulnerable.

But if even a newspaper as pretentious and worthily dull as the *Independent* was trying to court popularity, then there is a lesson for all of us.

Every quarter someone (I don't know who, some anonymous benefactor who thinks I should be bettering myself) sends me the widely respected and academically impeccable *Drug and Therapeutics Bulletin*. As I am Sometimes A Good Doctor, I read it, though I usually skip straight through to the conclusion.

I suppose this is cheating, but it's not an inviting read. Its very appearance bespeaks gravity and austerity: no photographs, no colour, no poetic exaggeration, no leavening of humour. If it had been required reading for the Spartan children on their overnight ordeal on the mountain, most of them would have reneged and headed for

Ibiza to chill out and smoke lotus petals. It is unfailingly cold and logical, the Mr Spock of medical journals.

Even the conclusion is tough going: dry and academic, every objective assessment cogently and impeccably argued, but I do wish for a bit more passion, more Bones McCoy than Mr Spock. We are not robots, not automatons, and we respond to the heart as well as the head.

"The best lack all conviction, while the worst are full of passionate intensity," said Yeats, and we see this dichotomy all over the globe and all through history. But why in medicine; why should we cede the passionate intensity to the charlatans? We need more ferocity, we need the rage to win, we need the rough beast.

If the *Drug and Therapeutics Bulletin* is right, and it always is, its message should be throbbing with righteous wrath, and appeal to the emotion as well as the intellect. I'm thinking something like "Mandy is 22, enjoys dancing, shopping and dwarf-smuggling, and wants to work for world peace and marry a footballer.

"And she thinks that this new non-steroidal anti-inflammatory is shit."

Medicine is not a club

BMJ 6 April 2006

There is a small hospital in Drogheda in Ireland, where, between 1974 and 1998, 188 peripartum hysterectomies were performed, most of them caesarean hysterectomies, and most by the same doctor; most obstetricians would carry out less than 10 in their whole career.

That a doctor should deviate from normal practice is not exceptional; we can all get set in our ways, and nowadays change occurs so rapidly that it is easy to fall behind. But in this case the practice adopted at the hospital was so unusual that surely it should have been noticed. The other obstetricians, the midwives, the anaesthetists, the paediatricians, the registrars, the physicians, the surgeons, the local general practitioners, surely one of them should have noticed that something was going on. And yet the Royal College of Obstetricians and Gynaecologists inspected the unit as recently as 1992 and found it suitable for training.

A complaint was eventually made (courageously, it must be said) by a newly appointed midwife, who obviously didn't understand that rocking the boat was not what the doctor ordered. This complaint was then investigated by three Irish obstetricians, who found that there was no case to answer.

A later and highly critical government report dismissed this finding as motivated by "compassion and collegiality," and this is what I find most disturbing. Who most deserved the compassion, the obstetricians' colleague, or the women who had this unnecessary procedure, with all its implications?

And what does "collegiality" mean? It implies a "them and us," that doctors and patients are mutually exclusive groups. But they aren't; every one of us will be a patient sooner or later.

We are slow to criticise each other because we understand that humans are frail, that mistakes are easily made, and that we could be the next to make one; we don't want to cast the first stone. We also know that often bad things happen and it's nobody's fault, that we manage uncertainty every day and sometimes the gamble comes unstuck, that medicine has its limitations and that patient expectations are often unrealistic.

But none of these should translate into a misplaced loyalty to our profession when we can see that something is clearly going wrong.

When I became a doctor, I didn't join a club.

Beware of awareness weeks

GP 25 April 2014

I am sceptical about awareness weeks. The very last people to benefit are the patients. Instead, vested interests masquerade cunningly as advocates of the public good. The pressure group or charity is keen to show it is actually doing something. The PR firm is delighted to soak up funds raised by raffles, marathons, charity walks and sponsored head-shaves. There's often a pharmaceutical company in the background, eager to raise public anxiety about an illness for which it conveniently sells products.

So I've come up with a few ideas for some more realistic awareness weeks:

1. 'You're better off not knowing you're sick because there are no good treatments anyway' awareness week

2. 'If you think you feel bad now, just wait till you get the treatment' awareness week

3. 'There is actually nothing wrong with you' awareness week

The snake oil salesmen will never miss an opportunity, so surprise, surprise - as I write, it is Homeopathy Awareness Week. This is all right with me, as long as the awareness raised is that homeopathy is nonsensical, peddled by charlatans hiding behind an illusion of knowledge. Though as alternative medicine goes, it's not the worst. Compared with traditional Chinese medicine, which is contributing to the imminent extinction of the tiger and the rhino, homeopathy's downside is pretty mild.

Grudgingly, I admit homeopathy does have a social conscience. There is an organisation called Homeopaths Without Borders, a non-profit organisation whose mission is 'to provide humanitarian aid, homeopathic treatment and education as partners with communities in need'.

Which essentially means it goes to nations with substandard healthcare and dilutes it even more to make it 10 times as good as healthcare in wealthier nations.

Less *Medecins Sans Frontieres* and more *Medecins Sans Medicine.*

Health promotion; a sacred cow

GP 13 September 2016

'I'm here for health promotion, I read about it in the paper. 'See your GP', it said,' said Joe.

'FFS, you were only here yesterday,' I said. He scowled in reply; there, you see, our conversation had only begun and I'd already made him unhappy.

We are doctors; we do terrible things to people. They come into the surgery like healthy folk and go out as patients. If they're really unlucky we confine them to an institution where the occupants are routinely left immobile, deprived of sleep, fed a diet that is tasteless and nutritionally marginal, and experience the de-humanising indignity of being half-naked all the time.

It doesn't have to be this way; the average age of a patient in general practice is 75. Many have multiple diagnoses, and their care is incredibly complex, and above all requires more of our time. But our time is in increasingly short supply, so much of it wasted on the worried well and on health promotion.

Health promotion is a sacred cow; it's so obviously a good thing, beyond reproach, how can you argue against it? Every few years a health minister comes out with the 'free health-checks, frcc MOTs!!' mantra, which makes a good political sound-bite but has minimal evidence base, takes up huge amounts of resources, and leads to vast amounts of bureaucracy and paperwork.

The human body is not a machine, but a complex, ever-adapting system. Keeping such a entity in good shape might seem a correspondingly complex task, but the essentials are not complicated; eat a balanced diet, take regular exercise, don't smoke, don't drink excessively. It's not rocket science, the message is clear and simple, so why it should take up so much of our precious time is unclear.

Of course, just because health promotion is simple, doesn't mean it's easy; the world is full of fleshpots and hedonistic distractions, and it's up to governments to enable and improve access to healthy lifestyles.

But it shouldn't need a consultation from us; we have sick people like Joe to look after.

Chapter 8

Christmas and New Year

Christmas means different things to different people. To ordinary folk it means tinsel, Santa Claus, carols, the horns of elf-land faintly blowing, good fellowship and hot, roaring fires.

But for family doctors time is artificially stretched; patients seem to think that Christmas lasts for about six months, during which time the health centre will be locked tight, which leads to things like the Christmas antibiotic (just in case, you understand) and the pre-Christmas check-up.

For us, it's more likely to be hot, roaring patients...

Humbug

BMJ 22 December 2001

I love Christmas. I love the carols, the companionship, the coldness, the friends coming home, the hot whiskeys and iced beers, the innocence, the magic . . .

But I love it too much. Like the smell of coffee or the prospect of making love to a beautiful woman, it can never live up to expectations, and you always need a smoke afterwards, maybe a cup of coffee.

Instead of my beautiful fantasy, what we have is a tawdry commercial extravaganza, trinkets in the shops from October on, PA systems in shopping centres relentlessly churning out 'Merry Xmas Everybody.'

It's all bollocks. All those little Nativity scenes on Christmas cards, Mary surprisingly fashionable in a deep blue gown, a rather elderly Joseph seemingly resigned if a bit depressed, the lighting soft and cosy as if there is a neat little campfire somewhere, the straw as inviting as a feather bed, the immaculately groomed animals looking benignly on.

But have any of you ever been unlucky enough to be in a stable on a cold December night? My Uncle Paid kept a few cows, mostly just to annoy me, I reckon, so I have tasted of that particular bitter cup.

A stable in winter is as uncomfortable as it is possible to be; cold, damp, dirty, mucky, there is a stink of sweaty animals and cow dung, the straw is both wet and itchy at the same time, and if you could light a fire, even with the straw being soggy the place would go up in flames before you could say 'J. ... C..., put that match out,' and the whole Nativity family would have been torched instantly and history taken a different course.

Even the giving and receiving of presents is flawed. We like to think that Christmas gifts from our patients are a symbol of generosity and gratitude, a sign that our relationship is not purely cold and professional, that the care we give to them comes from our hearts. But I have a salutary little parable.

Last Christmas an art student who I'd been counselling for a billion years brought me one of his paintings, in appreciation of all my help. I was very touched and thanked him sincerely.

And then, in the true spirit of Christmas, he said: 'I can get you a good deal on a frame.'

Tit-les

BMJ 20 January 2005

'It's The Tit,' said my receptionist, 'Merry Christmas.'

The Tit's party piece was to collapse at every local festivity. His nickname, I emphasise, referred to the tiny moustache affected by all male members of his clan. In a delightful etymological quirk, these moustaches are known colloquially as tits, ergo the Tit Magees. My patient had become head of the clan by outliving the rest, ergo The Tit. Titles are rare in this republican heartland; instead of Lords and Ladies, we have Tits (and Doctors).

When I arrived, The Tit was lying in the rain, a vast muddy heap, surrounded by the traditional crowd of adoring acolytes. I asked him if he could stand up. He smiled beatifically and belched helpfully in my face; The Tit had a simple way of expressing himself, never using two words where one eruption of bodily gases would do.

'Take him into my house,' said a woman, indicating her front door, only yards away.

'No,' said another bystander, 'I'm his sister and I live in the next house,' and I thought, hey, if it's just the next house...

So I assembled a squad of volunteers, six strong men and me at the head (somebody has to delegate, I wasn't shirking the physical aspect of family practice). I still seemed to be bearing most of the weight; The Tit had a huge head.

We reached the next house and his sister said, 'No, I meant the next house.' So we staggered past the next house, and the next...

At last, the sister directed us up to a front door which, I noted with fatal satisfaction, was too narrow. Halfway through we got, ending up with The Tit wedged in the doorway, while the crowd, which had followed us like a pack of wild dogs, watched in goggle-eyed fascination to see what further mayhem would ensue.

Eventually frustration lent me strength, and I grabbed The Tit by two of the many folds in his neck, wrestled him into the front room and levered him on to the couch with a passing forklift.

His sister came in.

'Isn't it a lovely time of year,' she said happily, and my cynicism was disarmed.

The Tit belched again, and a cheesy, yet curiously Christmassy aroma graced the air.

What Child Is This?

GP 17 Jan 2008

It will soon be Christmas again; Santa will be shimmying down chimneys in defiance of his unhealthily high body mass index, and on Christmas morning, homes all across Ireland and Britain will echo to hundreds of little voices crying, 'Is this all I got?'

Humbug; patients coming in mid-month for 'their' cert; low back pain, for four weeks, thanks, plenty enough to see them comfortably into the New Year, lots of free time to do their Christmas shopping and then put their feet up in front of the TV.

'Merry Bloody Christmas,' I'd snarl, folding the cert into a paper plane and throwing it at them, hoping to maybe hit them in the eye, if I was lucky give them a corneal abrasion, something to cry about over the holidays.

So rather than continue to endure such an annual disappointment, I turned my back firmly on the festive season. I was on a one-in-two night rota and Christmas was nothing but a prolonged torture, a succession of long winter nights, all the time acutely aware that normal people were out enjoying themselves and that I was a mug.

Sometimes the local church choir would come around, flogging videos, mugging immigrants and singing carols and collecting money for Sister Eucharia's hernia operation; 'Get out of my face before I hurt you', I'd say kindly, though in the end I'd relent and give them the traditional prescription for antibiotics, what with it being Christmas and all.

Then, one Christmas Eve, something strange happened. There was a knock at the door, and when I answered I saw a middle-aged man with a magnificent beard and a 'why me?' expression on his face, a very very very young woman sitting on a donkey, a squad of shepherds and three old guys with big parcels under their arms.

In general practice you have to be ready for anything; I'd read the book, I knew the score.

'There's a stable out the back, plenty of straw, no smoking please, a few appropriate barnyard animals, not too much manure, should suit you nicely,' I said.

'That's not why we're here, doctor,' said the bearded man, 'The Child is pulling at His ears.......'

Make Christmas Great Again

GP 15 December 2016

It would have been easier to ignore blood in my urine.

'For the last time, sod off and get out of my face,' I said. 'You're not getting any more sleeping tablets or sick certs and I'm not signing any more of your jury duty exemptions.'

The carol singers halted their rather cheesy version of *Have a Cheeky Christmas* (it had none of the grandeur of the original), looking rather disappointed.

'You're very cranky tonight, doc,' said one.

Yes,' I said. 'If only I had a reason.'

Unusually for carol singers, there seemed to be a lot of torches and nooses and pitchforks and fairy lights (in a tasteful swastika design), even a few shotguns, thought admittedly these were gaily festooned with tinsel.

'Another great Christmas tradition gone,' they grumbled to each other, 'God be with the old days.'

'What'll be next?' said one, 'No more nativity plays?'

'Or Christmas Trees.'

'Or buying lots of shit that people don't want or need.'

'Or dousing an effigy of your GP with petrol and setting it on fire, and sitting round the blaze telling stories and roasting chestnuts.'

Things got worse; of course they did, this being the era of Brexit and Trump and Boris and fear and xenophobia and intolerance.

'Or discriminating against homosexuals on religious grounds.'

'Or Christmas just-in-case antibiotics.'

There was particular support for this complaint.

'Yeah,' said another. 'You need the Christmas antibiotic, because the surgery will be closed for, like, two whole days; anything could happen.'

'It's the immigrants,' someone said. 'They're taking all the antibiotics.'

Someone passed around a plate of mince pies and sausage rolls; it takes more than an invasion of Polish mechanics and Syrian refugees to put carol singers off their food.

'I blame the EU,' said another. 'When Brexit finally happens, only people that deserve them will get antibiotics.'

There was brief silence, unless you counted the occasional pungent belch, as the crowd considered this, mentally dividing the universe into the deserving and the undeserving, and placing themselves on the appropriate side.

'After Brexit, Christmas will be great again,' someone said.

'Bigly great,' they all agreed.

Santa and de-prescribing...

GP 3 January 2014

In the Spirit of Christmas, I've asked Santa to slip down the chimney and steal all the old ladies' tablets. It spares the rest of us a perilous task; as the old saying goes, never get between a she-bear and her cubs, or an old woman and her tablets.

From watching the National Geographic channel, it seems whole economies have been based on the ability of little old women to carry huge loads on their backs, so we know they are pretty tough.

It's not all their fault, I admit, we GPs prescribe the stuff in the first place. When I was just a young buck on the wards a little old lady was admitted in a very drowsy state. She was taking multiple meds - hypnotic, sedative, antidepressant, H2 blocker, calcium supplement, vitamins (whichever was top of that week's hit parade), antihypertensives, glucosamine, aspirin, paracetamol and, of course, a laxative, as some conventions must always be observed.

We were outraged; what was the GP doing? Was he trying to kill this old lady? We self-righteously stopped all her medications and, gratifyingly, over the next few days, she began to revive. However, as she revived, we encountered the Catch-22; she also became aware her tablets had been stopped and commenced a war of attrition to reclaim them.

We resisted, of course, we were young and passionate and wanted to change the world, but she was remorseless, and gradually we gave in ... first a sleeper, then an antihypertensive, then the vitamin, until soon she was on the whole regimen again, with a few more going nowhere just for show (we were the medical ward and had to do something to prove our brio).

However, the wise GP can exploit even this most unholy desire.

Mrs Maguire was ailing, surrounded by anxious family, her condition undiagnosable to the inexperienced doctor, but she and I were old sparring partners and if I didn't know the cause, I certainly knew the cure.

'It must be the tablets,' I said. 'We'll stop them all and see what happens,' I added, then watched Mrs Maguire explode miraculously off the couch.

'Only joking,' I said.

A doctor is a man's best friend

GP 10 January 2017

To paraphrase W. Somerset Maugham's advice on writing novels (again), there are three ways of refusing Joe a prescription; unfortunately, nobody knows what they are. So as the New Year dawned, Joe arrived with the traditional shopping list of medications. Resigned, I was filling in page 1 (of 4), when he surprised me.

He leaned closer (I was backed against the computer and could recoil no further); my keen investigative instinct informed me, for once, he hadn't had curry for breakfast. Also, and this was really weird, I noticed that he'd moisturised.

'I was thinking,' he said. 'Maybe all these tablets aren't a good idea, that I should start an exercise programme instead. Which would you think is better?'

It was like asking, which would 1 prefer; silk or pubic hair? But I was silent for a moment; sometimes silence can be eloquent, and this silence was making a passionate speech that the chances of Joe making lifestyle changes was the same as a vulgar, uninformed narcissist becoming President of the USA...

The silence grew louder, and more disbelieving.

'Honestly, doc,' he said. 'I don't want any more tablets; I'm going to take up the bike, start taking exercise.'

This was a kind of psychic earthquake; plaster didn't actually fall from the ceiling, but it was close, like hearing the Darkling Thrush; 'At once a voice arose among/The bleak twigs overhead/In a full-hearted evensong/Of joy illimited.'

'I'm still young,' he continued, his voice soft, a troubled look in his eyes. 'I'm suddenly realising that these are my golden hours, but that all things must end. Our ultimate future holds only loss and death and decay, and with each passing year the grave yawns a little wider.'

I was ashamed of my cynicism; at this crucial time, Joe needed the support of his friends. And if, like Joe, you don't have any friends, a doctor is the next best thing.

There was only one possible solution; my duty was clear.

'Get back in your pod, you alien,' I said. 'I want my Joe back.'

Chapter 9
Fantastical adventures in family practice

There are no restrictions on coming to see a country doctor; you don't even need to be sick. So just about anything can walk through that surgery door; from the most sublime love story to the most sordid peccadillo, from the unutterably trivial to the unbearably tragic, from funny stories to little morality plays. After thirty years in practice nothing surprises me anymore, except maybe consultants actually returning my phone calls.

The good, the bad, the repulsive, these encounters are all part of the arcane lore of country practice, and I'm almost sure they really happened.

A conversation with the Great Doctors
BMJ 8 Nov 2013

We stand on the shoulders of giants, but it can be an uncomfortable perch.

'This will help your cough,' I said firmly, summoning up all the authority of our ancient profession, of our eternal battle against superstition and ignorance, of titans like Harvey and Lister and Semmelweiss and Pasteur, and of the sacrifices they made often in the face of persecution and ridicule.

'Simple linctus 10 mls qid,' I wrote, and the ghosts of the titans shrank back in disgust. Lister made a retching noise, and Semmelweiss gave me the fingers.

But what can I do, I asked. There is a long cultural tradition of prescribing bottles. The placebo effect may be significant; it's a gesture of concern, that I'm taking the problem seriously—and it's safe: 'first do no harm' and all.

The ghost of Galileo appeared, waving his bloody thumbs at me. 'Look at these bad boys,' he said bitterly. 'The fucking pope did that to me, and I endured all this torment for what?'

'Some bastards even tried to poison me,' chipped in Galen. 'And for you to prescribe sugar flavoured water is spurious and deceitful. A Cochrane review of the use of antitussives in patients with acute cough showed no clear benefit for duration of cough.'

'That's pretty rich,' I said, 'coming from someone whose anatomical knowledge was gained from dissecting monkeys.'

'That's true, monkey boy,' said Vesalius. 'You proposed that that the interventricular septum was permeable; set the science of anatomy back a thousand years.'

'Hey,' said Galen, 'they wouldn't let me use gladiators; I tried it once and then there was all this 'I am Spartacus!' shit.'

By now I was feeling like a Fox News anchor, and getting sick of all this, like, science. Climate change denial, creationism: at last I understood the attraction, the simplicity of it all. Science is just too conflicting and confusing; fantasy is safer.

'Confusion is not an ignoble state, lad,' said kindly old Bones McCoy, 'Sometimes there's no right thing to do, just the least wrong thing; that's real medicine for you.'

'Remember,' said Van Helsing, 'a firm stab, through the heart.'

'Surely you can't be serious,' I protested.

'I am serious,' said Rumack, 'And don't call me Shirley.'

The first recorded case of Childhood Obesity

BMJ 18 Mar 2013

Finding the Magic Cottage was tricky. I asked directions from a sulky young girl in a red hoodie. 'Get lost,' she said, 'I'm morphing awkwardly into adulthood. Subtext too subtle for you?'

I summoned the great god Pan. He was adjusting his loincloth, which was revealingly and impressively askew. 'Sorry, can't stay,' he smirked, 'A wood nymph just called around; comprendez?'

I eventually tracked down the cottage by the pricking of my thumbs, and judicious use of sat-nav. Reality was on holiday, shacked up somewhere with the laws of physics. The front door smelt of gingerbread, and I noted the many multi-coloured mushrooms in the garden, all with their own tiny little doors and windows.

I tried the doorknob, which was made of chocolate and wouldn't turn properly. 'Even fairyland must have its laws,' said GK Chesterton, to which he might have added, 'and it ain't immune to shoddy workmanship either.' I pushed on through, treading on an inattentive pixie, the gingerbread door crumbling a bit, my feet sticking unpleasantly to the marshmallow carpet.

It was your average magic cottage—ancient crone, cookie-dough furniture, a couple of goblins molesting a squirrel—except for an expensive flat screen television and Sky box.

'Sure you're a real witch?' I asked suspiciously. She handed me a certificate. 'Member of the Royal College of Witches and Chiropractors,' it stated.

'Unbelievable,' I said.

'Yeah,' she said, 'Even fairytale creatures know chiropractic is a crock of ....' She stopped.

'Oi, you!' she shouted out the window, 'Scram, or I'll set the dogs on you.'

'That Terry Pratchett again,' she explained, 'Always snooping round.'

Two really fat kids lounged on an Ikea settee, stuffing themselves with doughnuts as big as my head.

'I'm worried about Hansel and Gretel's weight,' she said.

'Plenty of exercise, a balanced diet ....' I began.

'No, doctor, you don't understand,' she said, 'I need to beef them up, poor little things. Look at them, they're wasting away.'

Hansel belched loudly in agreement.

'What have you been feeding them?' I asked.

'The very best,' she said, 'Home cooked, organic, and all.'

I lifted a supersize McDonalds Happy Meal wrapper.

'So what's this?' I accused.

She looked embarrassed: 'The new cooker was being installed, so we had to order in.' The traditional oven, I noted, had been replaced by an enormous Aga.

Cometh the hour, cometh the doc; stories have their own atavistic power, and I understood my obligations.

'Very country kitchen chic,' I said, 'Show me how it works.'

House proud, she bent down to twiddle the knobs. I shoved her inside and, in tribute to Spinal Tap, turned it up to 11. Build a witch a fire and she's warm for a day, throw her in the fire and she's warm for the rest of her life.

At least we won't need the Liverpool Care Pathway, I thought.

Conversations with a pill

BMJ 2 January 2013

'You don't appreciate us,' he lamented, sitting on the edge of the desk, little legs dangling in the air. 'No thanks, just complaints about dependence, cost, side effects. 'For when the noble Caesar saw him stab, Ingratitude, more strong than traitor's arm, Quite vanquished him; then burst his mighty heart.''

'Think about it,' he continued. 'We are convenient, easily transported, eminently suitable for use in the home. Our quality can be monitored, standardised, and regulated; our dosages are reliable and flexible, we're uniquely suited to testing in double blind, randomised controlled trials. We're hardcore science, Student T-Tests, significance levels, chi squares; evidence-based medicine at its finest, none of this fuzzy holistic shite.'

'Providing the trial results are released, even if the results are negative,' I said.

'Of course,' he said.

'And made available to peer-reviewed journals,' I said.

'Goes without saying,' he said, 'Been following Richard Smith and Ben Goldacre on Twitter, have we?'

'You have to admit,' I said, 'your record is a bit dodgy.'

'Can't argue with that,' he shrugged. 'Statistics are sluts; for the right money, they'll prove anything you want them to, and drug companies are greedy, blood sucking, capitalist pigs who will be first against the wall when the revolution comes. But that's what makes the world go round, man.

'Greed is good, alas,' he said. 'Profit is the motivator, the innovator; if the pope or Mother Teresa ran a drug company, would any new products be developed? I'm small, not cheap.'

'And vitamin pills and homeopathic pills and flower remedies?' I asked.

'Yeah, yeah, a load of shite, I know,' he said. 'But everyone has relatives they ain't proud of.'

He drew himself up.

'We are of ancient provenance,' he said, and for a moment his voice sounded far distant, heavy with longing and loss, his little head hanging low, 'And across the ages we have wedded ourselves to humanity. We hitched our wagon to a star, but when the last human breathes his final breath under the indifferent skies, we will die too.

'Why do you need us so much? To paraphrase Tolstoy, the strongest of all cures are these two, time and patience; but humans have no patience.'

'I'm going to eat you now,' I said.

'*Et tu, Bruté*?' he said sadly. 'Then fall, Cialis.'

Footnote; you'll need to google Cialis…

Count your blessings….

BMJ 4 Jan 2003

'Ah, the children of the night …'

'Yeah yeah, what beautiful music they make yaddyaddy-adda,' I said, sitting well away, not from concern for my personal safety (a family doctor should never show fear), but when your diet is fresh blood, your breath stinks. 'I'm a busy man, Count, skip the theatrics.'

'I am in a most grave predicament,' he said, in a rich deep voice, which would be ideal for flogging complementary medicines. 'This warfarin—so many of my clients are taking it now that it is causing me considerable distress.'

'There, there,' I said, because even the undead deserve counselling, 'tell me about it.'

'I bite the neck, the blood flows, I lap it up with eager tongue, the blood clots, I stop. So it has always been. Now the bleeding does not stop, the blood is everywhere, up my nose, on my dress shirt—do you know how expensive these things are nowadays?—and I am a vampire, if I see blood I must drink of it. I even bring along a first aid kit, stick on a little bandage to stop the bleeding.' He gave an embarrassed, mournful shrug. 'Yet still I am putting on a little weight.'

'You aren't comfortable with your body,' I observed, with a Freudian insight, 'hence the big castles.'

'I don't feel good about myself, doctor. The ladies, they used to love me, they would lie there in those come-to-bed nightdresses, the intoxicating scent of garlic filling the air. I love garlic, you know, it's a little joke of mine.' A wintry smile broke through, then his tone briefly became sharper: 'This is confidential—right?'

'Of course,' I said.

'Ah,' he whispered, sad again, 'how they would scream, how they would moan with rapture, and next morning pretend they remembered but a nightmare. Now they scream only because I am become so fat I am squashing them. 'Get off me, Porky,' said one.

216

'And it gets worse: when I transform into a bat, I am too heavy to take off, I flap and I flap and I flap but I remain squat on the ground; the children of the night, how they snigger and smirk at me. I now must climb the drainpipe, so undignified, what with the extra weight and all. Last night, the drainpipe came down; I got a pain in my chest, I'm breathless, and I'm having palpitations.'

I examined him; the irony was thick. 'Your pulse,' I said, 'is irregularly irregular ...'

Footnote; atrial fibrillation is an irregularity of heart rhythm. It is often asymptomatic, but does increase the risk of blood clots, so when detected, patients are usually started on an anti-coagulant drug such as warfarin. On examination, the pulse is typically irregularly irregular...

A Whale of a time

BMJ 13 Jun 2012

Things are not always as they seem. The earth is not flat, the sun does not revolve around the earth, Boy George is actually a boy, Afghanistan is not an easy place to invade, and the United Kingdom's NHS reforms are in fact castrations.

I was whale-watching in the west of Ireland. It was an almost idyllic day, as we drifted through the early morning sea mist among the shearwaters, watching stormy petrels dancing on the water. The silence was made even sweeter by the soft rumble of the engine, the gentle sussuration of the Atlantic swell, the retching noises coming from the landlubbers in the bow, and the sniggers from the rest of us. We were, as Evelyn Waugh said, full of the comfort that glows in the heart of men as they contemplate the misfortune of their contemporaries.

Except that we had seen no whales, and by this stage even Captain Ahab might have said, 'Blow this for a game of soldiers, I'm off to have a keg of rum and violate a few cabin boys.'

Then, a jubilant cry: 'There's something in the water—it's black and white!'

A killer whale, we all thought, instantly electrified. Even our taciturn skipper was excited, and he wheeled the boat around for a closer look. As we came closer, we caught tantalising glimpses; to quote Joseph Conrad, 'Men learn wisdom with extreme slowness and are always ready to believe that which flatters their secret hopes.'

'I can see a fin,' someone shouted, and our anticipation surged in crescendo. 'It's a dorsal fin; looks like an old male; they're more solitary, you know,' he added, quite the expert.

As if on cue, to crank up the tension even further, the shearwaters took off in a whirl of ocean spray.

Then a dead, very dead, black and white cow floated up to the boat; doing it's best to be threatening, it gamely butted at the hull, but gently, so as not to upset anyone.

The 'expert' poked at it hopefully with a stick, but it didn't respond or try to fight back; it was definitely a dead cow.

'Thanks for nothing, Fin-boy,' I said.

Just call me Ishmael

GP 13 February 2018

His wooden leg was causing him considerable distress, he said; it was constantly painful and restricted his mobility, making him irritable all the time.

I referred him to prosthetics; he was fitted with the latest plastic gizmo, and, liberated from the chronic discomfort, his demeanour was transformed. In no time he was scampering around the village, playing football with the kids and goosing the old ladies. He got married, settled down, opened up a barber-shop, and forgot all about his sworn vengeance on the Great White Whale.

I had not only removed his wooden leg, I had removed his motivation; less driven, less compelling, though much happier, Captain Ahab's gain was great literature's loss.

Our role as doctors is to care for everyone, young and old, rich and poor, native and alien, real people and those who are not. My reputation mushroomed, and the next day the waiting room was packed, heaving with … heaving bosoms and moral dilemmas.

And also, notably, a foul and pestilent congregation of vapours. I called in the source, a haggard and woebegone young knight, referred him to the respirologists, and advised an online dating service.

'La belle dame sans merci no longer hath thee in thrall,' I said.

Then a Ms Louise Alcott came in. 'Wipe that smile off your face,' she snarled, in a distinctly unladylike manner. 'Beth Marsh was here, wasn't she?'

I pointed out that medical confidentiality was all-encompassing, which included imaginary people.

'She had scarlet fever, and you just had to give her antibiotics,' she said. 'Thus preventing her from developing rheumatic fever and suffering a life of disability and an early death. My whole Little Women gestalt is superfluous; no self-sacrifice, no lifetime of selflessly caring for Beth. How are their characters expected to grow? Years

219

of hard work up the Swanee, thanks to you and your fucking antibiotics.'

Unfortunately, happy, healthy people do not make interesting characters. To develop and grow, we need a challenge, a conflict. Everything worthwhile that will ever happen to us will involve pain and distress and cognitive dissonance.

As Harry Lime said in *The Third Man*: in Italy under the Borgias they had terror and bloodshed, yet also Leonardo da Vinci and the Renaissance. In Switzerland, 500 years of peace led only to… the cuckoo clock.

A Classic Surgical Error……

BMJ 28 August 2013

'What is your opinion, Watson?' asked Holmes.

'Definitely dead,' I intoned with Solomonic authority, 'On account of his head being missing and all.'

Holmes turned the body over. The crowd gasped in horror; someone fainted at the back and a few skinheads went through his pockets.

'Observe the pattern,' he said, 'This victim, like the others, has had both a haemorrhoidectomy and a hernia repair.'

'So?' I said.

'So,' he said, 'I deduce that the serial killer is a general surgeon; no one else does those procedures anymore. They are much reduced; time was when the general surgeon was the prince of the medical world, had the biggest shiniest car, and would have a go at anything—hemicolectomy, aortic aneurysm repair, thyroidectomy—but their empire has been eroded by the subspecialists and by clinical oversight and outcome audits; that which they were, they are not.'

'And the motive?'

"Consider the long arduous years of training, with the promise of some far-off golden day being able to operate on big stuff, then being forced to endure session upon endless session of ligating varicose veins and excising lipomas and sebaceous cysts,' said Holmes, 'The mighty heart is cracked at last.

'Too long a sacrifice can make a stone of the heart,' I agreed.

Holmes extracted a document from the victim's pockets.

'A set of guidelines,' I said.

'Another sign,' said Holmes, 'A slavish devotion to following guidelines.'

'Yes,' I said sadly, 'There are guidelines for everything these days; even, I believe, guidelines for writing guidelines.'

'And according to those guidelines ...' Holmes searched the pockets again, and with a flourish, produced another document, 'Evidence of premeditation.'

'A consent form,' I gasped, 'Hell is empty, and all the devils are here.'

'Which,' observed Holmes, 'in a crucial error, typical of the egotism of the serial killer and the general surgeon ... the murderer has counter-signed.'

Co-lumbo, co-codamol, and co-nstipation

BMJ 28 Sep 2011

When Kojak walked out of the surgery sporting a magnificent mullet, word of my semi-miraculous skills soon got around to the other great detectives. Most of the cases were straightforward: Cannon was underweight (the camera is fattening), Batman had a rubber allergy, and Porfiry Petrovich had diarrhoea after a bad bowl of borscht.

But Columbo? It seemed an uncomplicated tension headache, so I gave him some general advice on lifestyle changes and a prescription for co-codamol. 'That's great, wonderful,' he said, 'thank you, doctor, thanks you, you've been very helpful.'

Then, at the door, he turned, with a swirl of his shabby raincoat.

'Just one more thing, doctor,' he said, 'A small thing; but it's been annoying me. Co-codamol: that's a combination of paracetamol and codeine isn't it?'

'Exactly, Lieutenant,' I said, in the patronising 'pride before a fall' manner demanded by cinematic tradition. 'Just to give it that extra punch; like the adverts, you know: zap! Kapow!'

'Yes, of course, you're right,' he said. 'But there are a couple of loose ends I'd like to tie up; nothing important, you understand. I was checking out codeine as an analgesic, and it seems the dose is 30 to 60 mg every 4 to 6 hours.'

'Yes,' I said uncomfortably, beginning to see where this was heading.

'Yet,' he continued, 'The dose of codeine in my prescription and in the adverts is only 8 mg.'

'Indeed,' I said weakly. 'For that extra punch, you know.'

'But 8 mg of codeine has marginal analgesic value.'

'Indeed,' I said, like a rat in a corner.

'Indeed yes or indeed no,' he asked.

'Yes,' I said wretchedly, breaking down at last and blurting out my confession, as is traditional, 'Okay, it's a fair cop, we use co-codamol because it sounds better than just paracetamol, which though undoubtedly effective, has suffered due to its ubiquity. It adds a bit of mystique and helps the placebo effect. Drug companies, I'm sure, share the same selfless motivation, and it's purely incidental that it makes them loads of money.'

'So, to conclude,' said Columbo, 'There are no advantages to co-codamol over paracetamol' (*MeReC Bulletin*2000;11:1-4R).

'Not exactly, Lieutenant,' I protested. 'Not if you enjoy being constipated.'

A Classic consultation...

BMJ 27 April 2011

Give a dog a bad name, said Flashy, it's far harder to live down a good one. So when the Greek heroes learnt that I had sorted out Heracles' bursitis, the waiting room was soon bursting with Homeric valour and atavistic rancor. The testosterone was sky high, an equal temper of heroic hearts and body oil, though we had to give the Trojans a separate room.

Some of it was predictable: Tithonus had dementia, and Polyphemus had glaucoma. But there was also the occasional surprise: Bellerophon was allergic to horse hair, and Oedipus was actually very kind to his parents.

Achilles came into the surgery, trailing a bored-looking Greek chorus. He squashed his mighty thews into the plastic-covered chair, which gave an amusing farting noise. Some members of the chorus sniggered.

'I usually see Asclepius,' he said. 'But it's always the same with him: 'Sacrifice Iphigenia here; libation to Apollo there; blah blah.'

'Trouble with the handmaidens again?' I asked; general practitioners are the Renaissance men of medicine; a knowledge of the classics is mandatory.

'No,' he said, 'I was racing a tortoise. Sounded easy, gave it a start, but each time I caught up it had travelled a small distance further. I was just about to overtake and disprove the infinity paradox when I tripped over a golden apple that Atalanta had left lying around. Now my ankle is giving me gyp. What about an x-ray?'

'An x-ray, an x-ray,' chanted the chorus.

I scrolled through his history.

'Ah yes, after your MMR vaccination, your mother dipped you in the River Styx, which made you invulnerable. This, incidentally, was the earliest recorded example of preventive medicine, and we were going to dip all our infants in there too, but then a paper in *The Lancet* suggested a link with autism. However, because she held you by the ankle, your ankle has no protection. But it's just a sprain. Rest for two weeks, and no slaughtering.

'And,' I continued, in a faux sepulchral tone, à la the Delphic oracle, 'don't go near the Scaean Gate.' Opportunistic health promotion is an integral part of the good doctor's consultation.

He looked concerned, obviously thinking about the handmaidens.

'Ravishing's okay,' I reassured him.

'Guess it could have been worse, doc,' he said, sounding relieved, 'At least she didn't hold me by the di—'

'Digits,' I said, pre-empting the chorus.

The Prophet of Nudge

BMJ 10 Mar 2011

'Life's not fair,' I raged. 'Why does god always take the smokers first?'

I was watching Joe's funeral. The church is inconveniently situated beside our health centre, and I usually duck out of sight as the cortege looks over accusingly.

But this time my conscience was clear: Joe had smoked like a chimney, and then, with cosmic irony, been hit by a meteorite.

But when God actually appeared to me I was underwhelmed. He was tall and rather pointedly Caucasian, with a long white beard - every cliché in the book, and, what's worse, he didn't sound one bit like Morgan Freeman. I stepped into the winged chariot, which was piloted by an angel. Male or female, I couldn't quite make out, but he or she was disconcertingly attractive.

'I have decided,' God said, a drum roll filling the air, 'to be more proactive on health promotion. The consequences of smoking will no longer be deferred; short term gratification versus long term punishment, with humans it's no contest. So I'm making it one of the Ten Commandments—I'll take out adultery; that's so 20th century. From now on, anyone who smokes is gonna get smacked in the face by a meteorite. Consider it a form of celestial Nudging.'

Nudge Theory argues that positive reinforcement and indirect suggestions can influence decision-making at least as effectively as direct instruction or enforcement, and is quite fashionable among our public health colleagues, who just love management stuff (far more than real medicine).

There was a squeak of annoyance, and the drum roll stopped abruptly as an angel dropped a drumstick over the edge of the chariot. It spiralled downwards into the clouds, nearly taking out a cruising US AWACS Hercules C-130.

'You shall be my prophet,' he continued, 'to spread the word of Nudging to the four corners of the earth.'

I looked at the other prophets doubtfully. They were smoking hookahs, foaming at the mouth, and torturing a pagan.

'I'll just put Nudging on Facebook and send out a few tweets,' I said (social media can be a great way of avoiding, you know, real work).

But I was getting the hang of the prophecy business; like any good American televangelist, there had to be something in it for me.

'Yea verily, Lord,' I said, 'I would crave a boon.'

'Seventy-six virgins wasn't meant to be taken literally,' he said, crooking a finger at an angel, who swayed toward me in a seductive yet non-gender specific manner. 'And,' he said, seeing my confusion, 'I'm making you bisexual.'

'Cool,' I said.

I'm a Celebrity doctor, get me out of here....

BMJ 19 Jan 2011

'I was once adored too,' says Sir Andrew Aguecheek, and with only those few words the clown's facade is ripped apart, and Shakespeare reveals a broken man, crushingly aware of his loss and of his decay into frivolity and irrelevance.

'I was once a celebrity too,' I say, and I also feel the loss - though the experience was not always pleasant. The camera is fattening, my bald head shone like a small sweaty moon, and in the publicity photos the diaphragm of my stethoscope hung down in a white blob at crotch level, looking like my zip was open and my jockeys protruding.

But once a media slut . . . 'We're planning a new series, *Celebrity Doctor*,' said the production company. 'Being a celebrity yourself, would you mentor a contestant?'

My immediate reaction, apart from being secretly flattered (we celebrities are deeply insecure and thus easily manipulated), was of outrage; to collude with this circus would be a slur on our ancient profession. These celebrities hadn't even sat the pre-medical aptitude test (for a mere £70), which shows how doctors are different from mere lay people; more ethical and compassionate, you know.

Then I had a magical thought.

'Could I have Stephen Fry?' I asked, indulging in a brief reverie, the great man and I engaged in scholarly banter by the fireside, perhaps writing a revue together, a droll spoof aimed more at the heart than the head; in revolutionary France we might have opened a salon.

'Yeh, good one,' they sniggered, 'But, seriously, we are talking Z-list here, weather girls, washed-up musicians, an actress who tried to lose weight by cutting her own head off, all shamelessly eager to be humiliated in any way as long as they get their picture in the tabloids. They need to be validated; we should stick nipples on the camera lens.'

'A persuasive argument,' I admitted. 'Because, after all, it's our vocation to care for everybody, even the completely deluded.'

'Yes, absolutely,' they brightened up; this was a loophole that obviously hadn't occurred to them before, 'That's right. These poor people need your help. Absolutely. It's absolutely your duty as a doctor.

'You'll tutor them for a few weeks, on the job training, and so on, then, bam! They do a surgery on their own. And we film everything, all the funny incidents, patients dying like flies, the emotional stuff.'

'Yeah,' I agreed, some ethical reservations rekindling. 'Patients dying like flies would certainly be emotional.'

Good/bad doctors and the Great Poets

BMJ 18 Apr 2012

'My heart aches, and a drowsy numbness pains my sense . . .'

'I get it Mr Keats,' I said. 'You're a bit depressed.'

' . . . and I feel like drinking hemlock, or some dull opiate emptying to the drains,' he said, a trifle sharply, as if annoyed that I had interrupted his flow. Hey, I'm a busy man, and at 6 to 10 minutes per consultation, just call me the GP from Porlock.

'Probably makes you want to jump on the viewless wings of Poesy,' I said, adapting quickly to the appropriate genre quickly; family doctors have to be able to do this kind of stuff. His eyes narrowed, and he furtively took out a pen and scribbled something down.

I was faced with a dilemma. His melancholic disposition was obviously the essence of his muse. Treat it successfully and I'd be depriving the world of some of the great works of English literature. The common good, said Pierre in *War and Peace*, is the only kind of good there is, but sometimes even good doctors just have to be bad.

Ever the alert clinician, I had also noted the lily on his brow and the fading rose on his cheek, so I reckoned we hadn't much time, which ruled out cognitive behavioural therapy and its billion-year waiting list.

So I gave him some general lifestyle advice: no more getting loaded on cups full of the blushful Hippocrene; the only beaded bubbles winking at the brim were to be from cans of Pepsi. Get out more, meet people, nix on the palely loitering. And you need more exercise, I said, a vigorous half hour's walk every day.

'And take time to smell the flowers,' I said.

'Smell the flowers?' he said, with a condescending smirk. 'What are you, one of those pre-Raphaelite bird-brains?'

I was reassured by this show of spirit, but as he had revealed a propensity to self-harm, I also started him on an antidepressant and arranged an early follow-up. Had I committed a crime, I wondered; would his literary genius survive my clumsy biochemical manipulations?

Two weeks later he returned.

'I wandered lonely as a cloud,' he simpered.

Forgive me, Melpomene, I thought.

The Quest...

BMJ *29 January 2004*

'I have a mighty task for you,' said Gandalf. 'The Dark Tower is rebuilt; orcs are multiplying like rabbits (they have no concept of responsible birth control), hobbits are being forced to get proper jobs instead of lying around drunk all the time, and flocks of confused and disoriented Nazgul are strafing Narnia with guano. The Dark Lord has awakened; he is seeking... The Ring.'

'What ring?' I said.

'This one,' he said, palming it from behind my ear. 'Though quite nice to look at, it corrupts the owner; they become hard and cynical and develop halitosis and crumbly fingernails.'

He took out a pipe and blew a magical smoke ring in the shape of a jewelled speculum.

'The elves have a saying,' he continued. ''When in doubt, call the GP,' and since ye are hard and cynical anyway The Ring can't make you any worse. It must be destroyed, and you must take it to the fires of Mount Doom, which inconveniently is right beside the Dark Tower; you may take any loyal assistant of your choice.'

'Could I have Lassie?' I asked.

'No problem,' he said, taking out a little book which was rather discouragingly titled *Easy Spells for the Young Apprentice*. There was a puff of smoke, Lassie burst joyfully into the room, snuggled into my lap and licked my hand, then tried to bite the ring and turned into a small, bewildered, drug rep who burst into tears, glad-handed us some promotional pens, and fled.

'Why not just hop on one of those big eagles?" I suggested. 'Fly down, chuck it in, and you'd be back before the Dark Lord could say, 'Galadriel is a cheap slut'.'

'Alas,' Gandalf explained vaguely, deftly pocketing the pens, 'Alack.'

'All right,' I said, 'I'll get rid of it.'

'The Seven Fairies shall sing your praises,' he said, getting up hastily to leave. 'By the way, can I have an antibiotic? I've an awful cou-...'

I closed the door firmly, accidentally crushing a dwarf, and eyed The Ring speculatively. Thin spidery writing appeared on it, ancient elvish runes, which roughly translated as 'Legolas fancies Aragorn.'

'From where I'm sending you, buddy, you ain't never coming back,' I said, popping The Ring in an envelope and addressing it to the local neurology outpatients.

And marking it 'non-urgent.'

'Knight' duty; a visit to the Lady of Shallot

BMJ 16 June 2005

'Tis the Lady of Shallot,' she said, 'Wouldst thou call upon me?'

'No chance,' I said, 'new NHS policy, not efficient use of time, etc etc.'

But she was a quick learner, knew all the tricks. 'I sense an ill humour, and central crushing chest pain radiating to my left arm and all.'

'Oh, all right,' I snarled graciously. Even fairy-tale patients know how to push our buttons and make us jump;

the university of the street could teach our medical students a thing or two.

I parked outside the tower in a temper, accidentally on purpose running over a unicorn (the presence of which would soon become clear). Stepping carefully over the equine haemorrhage, I followed a winding stair past the mural of Merlin catheterising The Green Knight. Rather nouveau riche design, I thought.

I tripped on some white glistening sticky stuff, of uncertain and possibly revolting provenance.

'Mind the web,' said a voice from behind a huge mirror, which I noticed was linked to external security cameras, 'it's a bugger to spin.'

'If I'm going to examine you, you'll have to come out,' I said.

'No man may look on me, else the curse come upon me and I perish.'

I drew myself up, feeling rather violated; 'I am not a man, madam, I am a doctor, and therefore an asexual mutant.'

A beautiful maiden appeared, garbed in voluminous white, a tad too Miss Havisham for my taste.

'Oooh,' she said, 'Aren't you the handsome young buck.'

My reflection in the mirror revealed a specky, balding person.

'Don't meet many guys, do you?' I said. 'Now, what about this chest pain?'

'I confess 'twas a mere contrivance,' she said, stroking my bald patch meaningfully. 'I grow lonely for male company and I figured, what the heck, GPs have to come out when you call, don't they?'

Her expression suddenly changed. 'I don't believe it,' she said peevishly, 'you wait a lifetime, and then two guys come along at once.'

On the camera screens I saw a knight in armour, brazen greaves glittering in the sun, his mighty stallion befouling the green sward in what looked like an annual catharsis.

'Gotta go,' she said.

I felt rejected; he was tall, handsome, and heroic, but I drive a Mercedes. Doesn't a big shiny car count for anything anymore?

Lancelot came running up the stairs, looking dashing if not very bright. His noble visage was grave and his eyes bugging out.

'Come quickly, Doc, the fair maiden…'

I noted with some satisfaction that his voice was nasal and squeaky.

'Yeah, I can guess, she's all a-swoon, is she?'

I checked her out; her chest was heaving prettily in the way only a very alert chest can manage.

'It's a bad case of melodrama,' I said.

No miracles in the NHS; a visit from Our Lord

BMJ 12 April 2007

'It's Our Lord,' said my receptionist, 'and before you ask, it's definitely Him, He has ID.'

'Hang on,' He said as He entered the surgery, 'I'd asked for a doctor that believes in Me.'

'Nothing personal, Lord,' I said, 'but to rational people You're slightly less believable than Santa Claus or homoeopathy, all that Samson and Goliath stuff.'

'Hey,' He said, 'Samson was a decent hardworking man; runs a barber shop now—or was it then?' He scratched his head: 'Omnipresence can be confusing, you know.'

'I'm feeling a bit depressed,' He continued, idly bringing my dead budgie back to life (I'd been meaning to get the cage cleaned out), 'Two thousand years, and very little gratitude; when things go well they take it for granted—when they go badly I get the blame.'

'Boy, could I sing a few bars of that,' I said. 'The real question is, just how depressed are You?'

'Oh, not too bad, I suppose,' He said gamely. 'So I thought . . .you know.... maybe a few tablets . . . '

'Alas,' I said, 'the latest guidelines from the National Institute for Health and Clinical Excellence (NICE) on mild to moderate depression are unequivocal. No medications for You, Lord; instead take plenty of exercise, eat a balanced diet, and try and get out some more.'

'What else do they suggest?' He said, visibly unimpressed by my lifestyle advice, further evidence of His human side.

'There's counselling,' I said.

'That sounds good,' He said, 'I'd like counselling. Where do I go?'

'Hey, we can put the show on right here in the barn,' I said, hoping a Mickey Rooney reference might cheer Him up. I patted Him on the knee and said, 'There, there.'

He seemed to find this unhelpful.

'Anything else?'

'Of course,' I said, 'Do you think the fine people at NICE are idiots, that they have no idea what's really going on out there, on the streets, with the kids? Cognitive therapy is a very effective treatment.'

'Great,' He said, 'I'll have some of that.'

'I have more bad news,' I sympathised. 'Because Your depression is only mild to moderate, You're not an urgent case. I can't refer You directly, You'll have to see a psychiatrist first, and non-urgent psychiatric cases are usually not seen for about six months, and the waiting list for cognitive therapy is another six months after that.'

'About a year in total,' He calculated, biting His lip. 'That's a long time to be depressed. Any other treatment options?'

'Nada, Zippo, Zilch' I said helpfully.

'Nada, Zippo, Zilch,' echoed the revivified budgie.

'So what NICE are saying, in effect,' He reasoned painfully, 'is that there are no treatments for mild-to-moderate depression.'

'It is You that say it, Lord, not me. Have a NICE day,' I said, getting up and washing my hands.

Footnote; NICE (the National Institute of Clinical Excellence) might be living on a different planet from the rest of us, but at least they have a sense of humour. Their chairman was most complimentary about this column.

Five go mad in family practice

BMJ 24 May 2007

Raised in rural Ireland, I used to read Enid Blyton just like everybody else, so a locum in the shires a few years ago was just like going home.

On my first morning the vicar waved to me in greeting, like John Major had promised, although I was then a bit surprised to see him slipping off his bike to trade Es with the local hoodies; things sure have changed on Walton's Mountain, I thought, but hey, that's the Church being more relevant.

And even more quintessentially English, that night I was called to the scene of a murder. The body was face down in the local cricket club, blood on his scalp, a bloody cricket bat lying beside him, and the assembled committee looking on with what seemed almost a sense of satisfaction and nostalgia, a glimpse of something they thought had been lost forever.

'And did those feet in ancient time/Walk upon England's mountains green?' murmured one old colonel reverently.

The policeman introduced himself as Constable Goode, and I felt I'd known him all my life.

'What is your opinion, doctor?' asked the constable.

'Seems dead alright,' I observed, facts at my fingertips, though my attention was distracted by a little old lady, scribbling furiously into a tattered old notebook; nosey old bitch, I thought.

'Excuse me, madam,' I said oleaginously (just in case she was someone important). 'Have we met?'

'Mrs Christie,' she said, which rang a few bells.

'Cause of death,' Constable Goode pronounced slowly, with the traditional air of intense concentration, writing in a little notebook with the mandatory stubby pencil, 'Trauma to head by person or persons unknown.'

I knew something was required of me, and I rolled the body over, squashing some egg-and-watercress sandwiches. The shirt had been ripped open, there were fresh bruises and burns on the chest, and the deceased had an annoyed expression on his face.

'Not so fast, sergeant,' I said (I always address coppers thus—a little bit of harmless flattery goes a long way), 'there's not enough blood. I therefore deduce that the head injuries were inflicted after death, as a cunning red herring.'

'A red herring?' mused the constable, 'in this plaice? Then what was the murder weapon?'

I pointed to the corner of the room.

'The defibrillator,' I shouted, 'J'accuse!'

The club secretary fell to his knees.

'OK, I confess,' he wailed. 'We've had that machine for five years, paid three grand for it. All those fund-raising garden fetes and sponsored walks and tea dances—if I ever see another cucumber sandwich I'm going to vomit. But in all that time we've never had a chance to use it, despite the publicity that people were dying like flies and about how important it was to have one; it's just been sitting there in the corner, laughing at us.

'So when Walter took a weak turn at the bar, we saw our chance; he fought bravely but we got him down in the end.'

Then a small curly-haired boy (or girl) popped her (or his) head round the door.

237

'Too late George,' said the constable, 'this case is closed.'

'F**** it,' said George, 'what'll I do with all this ginger beer?'

Footnote; When I was a child, there were no bookstores, no Amazon, so you read whatever books were available. I remember my dad buying a bookcase at an auction; the bookcase was full of books, Biggles, Enid Blyton, Gerald Durrell, Greek mythology etc. That was one very formative bookcase.

You think too much; survival of the fittest....

BMJ 5 July 2007

Having the great thinkers on your practice list can be a drag. The last time La Rochefoucauld came in, I happened to be reading a defence society magazine. 'There is something, Monsieur, in the misfortune of other doctors which is not entirely unpleasant,' I observed. His eyes narrowed thoughtfully, before launching into yet another long story about his sinuses and how dry they were (he preferred them pleasantly moist).

Hippocrates had just legged it from a foam party in the Groves of Academe and left the whole place soaking wet, and when Nietzsche was here he wouldn't wait in the queue like everyone else; we had to forcibly eject him by quoting Immanuel Kant at the tops of our voices. His complaint cited something about 'ubermenschen' and creating his own morality and not suffering the consequences of his own actions; and besides, all he wanted was an antibiotic because he had an awful cold and he had been fighting it himself for a week and it wasn't getting any better.

Darwin's inability to book an appointment proved just a minor obstacle to someone who spent 15 years studying barnacles. I was stopped at the only set of traffic lights in the village, when there was a rap at the window. I ignored it, but Edgar Allen Poe knew what he was talking about and you can't continue to ignore rapping evermore, plus the damn lights wouldn't change.

I resignedly rolled down the window, observing with fatal satisfaction that the red turned to green right on cue, so I switched on the hazard lights to warn the cars stuck behind me that this was going to take some time.

'I am concerned,' said the great man, 'about the direction of modern medicine. It is counterintuitive to the theory of evolution. You are perpetuating faulty genetic codes by artificial methods; maladaptive genes are being allowed to procreate; and the fitness of the human race is diminishing.'

'Maybe we are simply adapting rapidly to a new dynamic,' I replied, conscious of the honking horns and increasingly angry shouts behind me and trying to keep it brief, 'Maybe fitness is a broader, more flexible concept.'

The deep brow furrowed, the honking and the clamour grew more frantic. In my rear view mirror I could see a herd of cows charging up the road and thundering into the melee, body parts flying everywhere, like Pamplona with more dung but without the Iberian charm.

I hopped out of the car.

'Better run, Charles,' I said, 'It's survival of the fittest.'

239

Skippy's last show

BMJ 16 August 2007

I am laid back about emergencies; the little boy has cried 'WOLF!' once too often for me. Fax a photo of the wolf chewing on his scrotum, I say, and I might think about it. But the chains of our solemn office bind us tightly; when we are called, we gotta go, no matter how bizarre the circumstances.

One day a little kangaroo hopped into the surgery, making urgent chittering noises. I love wild creatures, so I reached for my gun; stuffed and mounted, I thought, it would make a nice trophy for the waiting room, maybe scare the kids a bit, keep them out in the fresh air and away from the health centre and all those superbugs.

'Wait, doc!' my patient shouted, just before I squeezed the trigger, 'He's trying to tell us something . . . something about a little girl, bottom of a cliff, broken leg, may need a splint, analgesia, and a drip.'

'Thanks for nothing, Dr Doolittle,' I said.

When we got there the mandatory crowd had gathered, and there was already a festive mood; multiple tinnies had been cracked open and someone had inflated a bouncy castle. A little blonde-haired girl, unmistakably and adorably Aryan, lay at the bottom of the traditional cliff. I noted, with a fatal satisfaction, that the cliff looked on the verge of collapse. Someone had inexplicably obtained a park ranger's uniform and was unsuccessfully trying to conceal his enormous enjoyment.

'Her leg's real crook, doc,' he said, 'you better get down there.'

I was in my good clothes, it was muddy; where were all those paramedics in combats when you need them, I thought.

Eventually I got down, signing a few autographs and reluctantly dismissing a groupie on my way; with so many watching, even a quickie was out of the question.

'It's a sprain,' I shouted up, and a ripple of fascinated horror went through the crowd; 'A sprain, a sprain,' they wailed.

'The copter's on its way, doc,' said the park ranger enthusiastically, 'but we'll have to MacGyver a stretcher from didgeridoos and wombat hides.'

'Actually, a sprain's not too bad,' I said, professional integrity outweighing the need to consummate the melodrama, 'Up you get, girlie.' A little pinch emphasised my authority and she got to her feet reluctantly. The crowd began to drift away, giving me disapproving looks; diverting from the original script was obviously considered bad taste.

Skippy reappeared: 'Something about a cave, a landslide, two kids, a pneumothorax, a chest drain, and . . . '

A single shot echoed through the eucalyptus groves, and far away a flock of parakeets rose, their wings golden in the sunset as the credits rolled for the last time.

Le Beau Doc Sans Merci

BMJ 24 November 2001

I met a young lady in the meads. Her hair was long, her step was light, her eyes were wild; she had intended to go to medical school, she said, but she had visited the local hospital and the junior doctors had discouraged her, and she was considering dentistry instead.

I set her on my pacing steed and all day long extolled the virtues of medical life.

'Asking a junior doctor what it's like to be a doctor is like asking a tadpole what it's like to be a frog,' I said.

'Consider being able to travel all across the world, the privilege of receiving the trust of our patients, the fascinating complexity and uniqueness of every case that walks into the surgery. Consider the security of tenure, a reliable income in a volatile world. Consider the independence; once you are a GP or a consultant, you are your own boss and you don't have to suck up to nobody. Ours is a high and noble destiny, a life rich with experience, an epic poem of joys and sorrows.

'We need a system of work experience for young people like you who are genuinely interested. It would be easy to determine which consultations are inappropriate for you to attend, and of course patients would be fully informed and consented. But even within these confines, it should be possible to get a taste of the real thing, and much better than learning from junior doctors or television soaps.'

The chill of icy air startled me from this reverie. We had stopped on a bleak hillside, ravens were croaking hoarsely, The Creature from the Black Lagoon was playing pinochle with an insurance salesman, and high overhead an American bomber was chucking out enough food aid to fill a small knapsack; the omens were bad. Sure enough, a tin of beans plummeted down like a rocket, nearly decapitating my horse, and my student became fey and magicked. She wove a circle round me thrice, her eyes flashing, her hair floating, gratuitously acting out the wrong poem.

'*La belle dame sans merci hath thee in thrall*,' she exulted, then turned into a chimera, then a gorgon, then back into a girl (with now rather frizzy hair) before continuing, 'And I'm sticking with dentistry, if you don't mind, no fucking expensive and pointless aptitude tests for that.'

'OK,' I replied, booting her off the horse, spooking a passing nut-laden squirrel as she fell, 'In that case you can walk home.'

Search for the hero inside...

BMJ 24 Mar 2010

'I love the smell of naproxen in the morning,' said the grizzled veteran, surveying the flames and inadvertently disclosing his day job as a pharmaceutical adviser. 'Smells of . . . economy—and bendroflumethiazide,' he continued, starting to ramble pointlessly, 'That's cheap and all, just the kind of drug a commie pinko would take. ACEs, ARMs, they're more the American way.'

Another fireman came dashing up.

'There are people trapped on the first floor,' he shouted at me enthusiastically. 'But you can't go in there: it's far too dangerous; you'd be risking your life.'

'Yes, absolutely, no problem,' I said. 'There are NICE guidelines for this kind of situation, which I cannot transgress. In case of fire, they clearly state, always take the advice of the experts. I'll just wait here then, shall I, while you chaps establish a perimeter, break down the doors with hatchets, get the hoses and ladders going, look macho, pose nude for charity calendars, and, you know, do your thing.'

The firemen appeared rather discomfited by this response. Briefly at a loss, they looked from me to the fire, then back to me.

'Don't even think about it,' said the first, gamely trying again, 'It's an old house made of wood, there's an oil tank in the basement, the roof is unstable and could go any-time, and the stairs are on fire and they mightn't bear your weight. It's a death trap.'

The crowd had seen it on television; they knew the drill. 'Don't go in there, you crazy fool,' they cried, 'You'll only get yourself killed; it's madness, you'll never make it out alive.'

The sense of expectation was suffocating, noblesse oblige and all that, and eventually I cracked, 'seeking the bubble reputation even in the cannon's mouth,' storming though the front door, racing up the stairs, heaving all available bodies onto my shoulders, stopping briefly to check my hair in a mirror.

'For a moment there I thought we were in trouble,' I dead-panned, then leapt out the window after accessorising with a convenient baby (for theatrical purposes), grabbed from an unqualified lay person. The crowd was ecstatic, and I handed the baby to a shadowy American Christian adoption agency, discreetly palming the fee.

'Look after the little mite,' I said, by now utterly in thrall to the stereotype, (and impressed by the fee), 'I gotta go back, there may be more babies in there.'

The posse; the male dream….

BMJ 14 February 1998

I wish I'd been a doc in the Old West; that was the life. A nice little house with a white picket fence, the respect of the hardworking but hospitable townsfolk, picnics with the buckboard, barn dances, hoedowns, scalp-hunting with John Wayne etc, etc.

And occasionally the highlight: the posse, the ultimate male bonding experience. Just picture it; stuck in a boring surgery when the sheriff runs in: 'Doc, the bank's been robbed.'

I'd git over there as fast as a horny toad on a hot griddle and see my buddies already saddled, in cracking form at the prospect of hanging out with the lads for a few days. There'd be a brief interlude of solemnity while the sheriff would swear us in as deputies, we'd get to wear a badge, someone would inevitably shout 'Yippi-eye-ay,' and away we'd gallop in the mandatory cloud of dust—if it was wet and muddy each man would have to bring his own dust—our body hair sprouting rampant even as we rode.

Being a doc, I couldn't be risked in the front line, so if any shooting started I'd be back at the chuckwagon with cookie, chewing tobaccy and waiting for casualties. These would usually involve shotgun pellets in the buttocks, which I'd remove in public under the anaesthetic cover of a slug of whiskey, accompanied by hoots of derision from the old-timers and admonitions never to stick your butt up in the air during a gunfight in case there's someone on the other side with a warped sense of humour.

And camping under the stars, spinning yarns, eating beans, and singing songs by firelight, like 'The girl I left behind me,' our eyes moist, our lower lips quivering, although inside we'd be thinking 'Hey; who needs her? Git along, little doggie!'

And sometimes in the night, all quiet except for those pesky coyotes, I'd be woken in a clandestine manner by the outlaw's trusty native American sidekick, Tonto Murphy (his mother was Irish).

'John-boy's been hurt bad,' he'd whisper, and my Hippo-cratic Oath would override my badge. Lancing his haem-orrhoid with a red hot poker, and dressing it with a hankie soaked in sweat, I'd find that he was a decent lad who'd fallen into bad company to support his sick Momma. I'd patch him up and promise to keep an eye on mom. 'Better mend your ways, boy, or next time I'll tan your hide,' I'd say in the appropriate gruff but kindly manner.

'Bless you doc,' he'd give the traditional reply, 'but now I have to smuggle some crack cocaine over the Rio Grande, so sod off.'

And as we'd ride back into town, the folks would flock to welcome us.

'There goes ol' Doc Farrell,' they'd say. 'He once shot a man in a fair fight, but it was over a woman and he came out west to forget; funny he turned out to be gay.'

Big tits

BMJ 11 January 2012

'Big tits,' agreed my colleague, enunciating the words with a certain relish, as it's not often we get a chance to say them with a clear conscience. 'Massive tits. The big-gest tits I've ever seen.'

We country general practitioners are close to nature, and we take our responsibilities seriously; we've kept a bird table behind the surgery for some years now. Birdseed, mealworms, peanuts; our menu is varied, but the favour-ite item is lard, and our generosity is now causing its own problems.

Give a man a fish and you feed him for a day, goes the proverb; teach a man to fish, and you feed him for a lifetime. Give a bunch of greedy little feckers a free lunch every day, and they'll stuff themselves until their tongues turn blue. We've enabled a handout culture, and reaped the whirlwind of gluttony and sloth.

As we watched, the biggest tit, engorged on saturated fat, flopped off the bird table, plopped on to the ground, and gave a few half-hearted flutters and squawks, before settling back with an apathetic shrug, as if to say: 'What can I do, it's not my fault, I hardly eat a thing, it's a hormonal problem.'

Health promotion is of prime concern to the diligent clinician, so I picked it up, took it in, checked its lipids, and gave it a lecture on diet and exercise. Fly, I said, be brave, sing your song, leap from tree to tree.

'Wheep,' said the tit, unenthusiastically. Couldn't you just give me a tablet or something, I could see it thinking.

I opened a window and set it free, to soar, I hoped, into the wide blue yonder. Unfortunately, I was on the second floor, and the tit dropped like a stone, stunning a passing climate change denier, before waddling determinedly back towards the bird table.

Less fat and carbohydrate, more fibre, I reckon.

And we're getting a cat.

Chapter 10
The Troubles

The Troubles were a terrible, sad time, so many lives wrecked and destroyed. And looking back, what was it all about, what was it all for, where did it get us?

Crossing the Border

Short-listed for the Michael McLaverty Short Story prize.

'Doc, we need you right now,' said the caller, in a hoarse voice I didn't recognise at the time, 'We've had an accident on O'Callaghan's farm; someone's been hurt, and it's pretty bad.'

'Right,' I said, 'I'll be over straightaway. I'll call an ambulance to meet me there-;'

I was interrupted. 'No ambulance, doc, just you,' and the line went dead.

I knew this had to be more than just a farm accident. The army were on the road in numbers, and on the way I was stopped at a checkpoint. They knew me; I'd attended the base the previous week after a mortar attack. Mortar attacks were a favourite local pastime when there was nothing good on TV.

'You're in an awful hurry, Doc. Where would you be off to?' asked the corporal.

'Sorry, can't tell you,' I said, 'Patient confidentiality, you understand. If I tell you, I'll have to kill you.'

The soldiers were even more on edge than usual, so something big had obviously happened. In the rear-view mirror, though, they didn't seem to be suspicious, just carrying as normal, shouting urgently into their radios and sending out carrier pigeons.

The farm was down a number of small boreens, winding in and out through the little hills of border country, tufts of grass growing in the middle of the road, a sign which usually precedes the twanging of banjos. When I arrived, everything was quiet, apart from the frenzied snarls of a chained guard-dog, but I knew I was being watched.

'Too quiet,' I thought, remembering my westerns.

There was no sign of any of the O'Callaghan family, and my knock was unanswered, so I went in uninvited, and in the front room I found James O'Connor lying on a couch, blood pooling on the floor beside him.

I'd known James for some time, and he had always seemed a studious, earnest young man. He'd been in Long Kesh for a year, which in retrospect had been no surprise. I had learned that the quieter and more discreet somebody was, the more likely they were to be involved. Volunteers rarely gave themselves away by talking too much or drawing attention to themselves. I'd heard that while in Long Kesh he was taking an university degree in English Literature, which also hadn't surprised me; republicans were well known for using their time at Her Majesty's Pleasure to further their education.

'Doc, I thought you'd never come,' he said, 'I've think my leg's broken.'

He was as pale as a winter's morning, and under a grimy woollen jumper his jeans were shredded and covered in dark red stains. I could see blood still seeping from his left thigh, though maybe not heavily enough to account for his pallor.

'Jesus, James, what happened to you?' I said.

'Gunshot wound, doc,' he said, 'among other things.'

I cut back his trouser leg; there was a deep wound on his left thigh and worse than that, it was bent and crooked, obviously a fractured femur. His blood pressure was low, his pulse was fast, real danger signs.

'James, we have to get you to hospital immediately,' I said, 'you're losing a lot of blood.'

He grabbed my hand.

'Not here, Doc, you've got to get me across the border, I'm not going back inside, not for anything.'

'James, you mightn't make it. The wound isn't as bad as it looks, but your leg's badly broken, and you're bleeding inside.'

I started dressing his wound, though the wound wasn't the real problem; the thigh-bone was fractured and the skin above it was becoming tense and swollen, indicating that an artery had ruptured and a substantial haemorrhage was going on underneath, unseen but lethal. He urgently needed the fracture stabilized, the artery repaired and the blood loss replaced.

I heard a noise at the front door.

James gripped my hand; 'Don't let them get me,' he whispered.

Part of me hoped that it was an army patrol, and my problem would be solved; James would be re-arrested and I could ensure he received immediate medical treatment.

'I'll tell 'em you've gone to the pictures,' I reassured him, 'You stay right here; and don't move.'

He laughed weakly, 'You're a real kidder, doc.'

Anton O'Carolan was standing at the door, middle-aged, medium height, stocky build, a carpenter with a reputation for few words and hard work. And, I realized, the voice from the telephone.

'I hear you have a casualty, Doc,' he said calmly.

'So you're connected as well, Anton,' I said, 'Another quiet man.'

'Those who speak do not know, those who know do not speak; Lao Tze," he said, deadpan.

We returned to the front room. 'What's to be done? Can we move him?' he asked

'I could tell you,' I said, 'but then I'd have to kill you; patient confidentiality, you understand.'

He nodded at James and received a thin smile in return.

'Tell him, doc,' said James.

'James needs hospital treatment. If he doesn't get it soon, he'll probably die. He'll be no use to the cause after that.'

'What do you think, James?' asked Anton, 'It's your call.'

'I'm not going back there,' he replied, 'No way, not ever.'

'There you are, doc,' Anton looked at me, 'It's up to you. You'll just have to do your best.'

'My best mightn't be enough, Anton,' I said, trying to make some sort of coherent plan, 'If he won't go to hospital here, we need to get him across the border and call an ambulance from there, and we need to do it quick. Bring the van up to the door, and make some room in the back, and I'll give him something for the pain and splint the fracture. And we'll need help to move him.'

'No,' said Anton, 'Nobody else needs be involved; no sense in more than the three of us getting caught.'

251

'Two of you,' I corrected him.

'Ah yes, of course, just two,' he said, 'I'd forgotten you weren't part of the armed struggle.'

'I have my own struggles, Anton.'

The van pulled off as gently as possible so as not to rock the patient. Due to the combined effects of the pain-killing drugs, blood loss and exhaustion, James had drifted off to an uneasy sleep.

'He broke out last night,' Anton said, 'it's been kept out of the news, but they've been hunting him hard ever since; hot on his trail since Whitecross, nearly got him up near Tullyvallen; that's where he was hurt. I could tell you more, but then I'd have to kill you.'

'It might have been better for him if he'd been caught,' I said.

'I know you don't approve of the armed struggle, Doc, but you haven't lived here long enough; you haven't had to put up with the discrimination, the persecution, being made to feel you were second class. You're a doctor, they don't harass you in the street and beat up your family and raid your house every few weeks.'

He was partly right; as doctors we were only bystanders at many of the tragedies and injustices, but I was too irritable to be apologetic.

'Look, Anton, I've been here long enough to see too many young lives ruined by the Troubles and by you and your armed struggle; you'd sit with scarlet majors at the base and speed glum heroes down the line to death. The rights and wrongs are beyond me, but we have another young life being ruined in the back of this van right now, and this one we could save. You're not bald or short of breath, but apart from that nothing changes.'

'Wilfred Owen,' Anton nodded, 'Very good. Doc; you should have been in the Kesh.'

'Siegfried Sassoon, actually," I said.

We pulled out of the boreen on to the main road and towards the border, barely a mile away. We had only turned the second corner when an oncoming car flashed its headlights at us, the traditional local signal that an army checkpoint was ahead. Anton pulled up immediately.

'We can't risk the car any more or they'll have us,' he said, 'We go on foot from here."

'Things keep getting better and better, don't they?' I said.

'You heard what he wanted, Doc,' he said.

'I heard a young deluded boy,' I said, 'It's rough country from here to the border. We can't carry him all the way; we'll have to wake him up, and it won't be pleasant.'

'Do whatever it takes,' said Anton, 'But make it quick; we'll have to go in a wide circle to avoid the checkpoint. They always have scouts.'

Anton opened the nearest gate and pulled the car into the field, tight in against the hedgerow for concealment.

'Real high-tech warfare, ain't it?' I said, 'At least it's a nice day.'

I shook James gently and he stirred and opened his eyes.

'Are we there yet, Doc?' he asked, like a child on a long car journey.

'Soon, James, very soon,' I said, 'But first we have to take a bit of a walk.'

He looked up briefly at hill in front of us, then closed his eyes; 'No problem, doc," he said, 'That which does not kill us makes us stronger."

'Not Nietzsche, please,' I said, 'Didn't they teach you anything inside? It'll be Kipling next."

'Nothing wrong with Kipling," said Anton, throwing a branch over the car, 'On the surface an imperialist sympathizer, but he understood the common man."

I took one arm, Anton the other, and we started across the field. The first half mile was easier, a gently sloping pasture under the shelter of the hedge of ash trees and wild rose. Then it began to get steeper, and the ground rougher, covered with wiry heather and scrub. We passed an army look-out post, one of the many that festooned the hills of South Armagh, but neither of us gave it even a glance. These posts were decorative only, rarely manned.

With every laboured step James would wince, and I was becoming exhausted myself. We finally approached the brow of the hill.

'Wait here,' said Anton, and he crawled forward, peering over the other side.

'It seems clear,' he said, 'let's go; we should be safe enough now. The border's only a few hundred yards away.'

As he finished a helicopter swept directly overhead, the rotors deafening, the mountain grasses whipping into a storm.

'Come on, we'll make it if we hurry,' urged Anton, but I could see that the down-slope was steeper, with deep beds of bracken to make the descent even more uncertain.

'We can't hurry,' I said, 'if he ever wants to walk again we have to take our time.'

He studied me thoughtfully.

'Right doc,' he said eventually, 'You're the boss; steady as she goes.'

We started down the hill, and by luck chanced on a beaten sheep-path through the bracken, slippery and only a few feet wide, but which meant that we could see where we were going. Not far ahead the bracken became more sparse and then merged into a more level field, and at the far end of that field I could see a gate.

'That gate's right on the border," said Anton, 'there'll be someone to meet us.'

'Nearly there, James,' I said, 'just a few more yards.'

A shot sounded, and I felt something whistle overhead.

'Get down,' shouted Anton.

'I can't get fuckin' down,' I said, crouching as low as I could, 'I'm holding James, if you hadn't noticed.'

'Yeah, doc, sorry,' he said, 'just acting on instinct; anyway, it was only a warning shot, they're quite accurate, you know, but let's get down just in case. And doc, please mind your language in front of the young lad.'

We laid James down as gently as we could and knelt beside him.

A loudspeaker hailed us.

'Stop where you are, we can see all three of you,' it said, 'Stand up and come forward with your hands in the air where we can see them, or we will shoot; this will be your only warning.'

255

I was almost relieved at this; in the thrill of the chase I'd lost sight of what was important and what wasn't. Escaping or not escaping was not relevant to me; I just didn't want my patient to die, and the sooner we were captured the sooner he'd get proper medical attention. I stood up with my hands in the air and waved as I'd seen them do on TV.

'Live long and prosper, Spock,' I shouted, making the appropriate hand-sign.

'We nearly made it, James,' I said, turning to him, but he wasn't listening. He was dragging himself hand over hand along the path down the hill.

'Stop it, you young fool,' I said, 'You'll never make it and you'll cripple yourself in the process.'

'I told you, doc, didn't I?' he hissed, inching forward, 'May as well bury me right here; I'm not going back inside, whatever the cost.'

I felt Anton's hand on my shoulder.

'The lad won't be taken, so you'll have to bring him, doc,' said Anton quietly, 'I'll hold them off.'

'This is madness,' I shouted at him, 'You're both gonna get yourself killed, and me as well, by the way, not that it matters or anything, I was having a bad day anyway.'

'That's the chance we all have to take, Doc, and anyway, you're as good as one of us now,' he said, smiling at me and pulling out and cocking a stubby revolver, 'Now you get going, and Doc?'

'Yes?' I said.

'Don't forget,' he said, 'Serpentine!'

'What's that?' I asked.

'I could tell you,' he said, 'but then-.'

'Yeah, yeah, then you'd have to kill me,' I said, 'Bullets really bring out your funny side, don't they?'

He bent down beneath the cover of the bracken and began crawling back the way we had come. Beyond him I could see small khaki figures scrambling over the crest of the hill and the helicopter approaching again.

'Don't worry, Doc,' whispered James, 'the 'copter won't come too close; we're too near the border, it might get hit by a ground-to-air missile.'

'Well, that certainly makes me feel much safer,' I said, 'Let's go, now it's just you and me, and, of course, the whole bloody British Army.'

We made slow stumbling progress along the path; after only a few yards I heard shouts from behind and a volley of shots ringing out. Would they shoot at us, I wondered, wishing that I had a little Red Cross flag I could hold up and wave in the air. We broke through the bracken; the going was much easier but now there was no cover. A herd of jersey cows had recently occupied the field and were now huddled in a far corner. I saw with a fatal satisfaction that they had left many large and pungent reminders of their presence, triumphant digestive mounds, and I made a mental note that when escaping across country with a wounded fugitive to in future I would choose a field without cows; sheep would be OK. A bullet tore up the ground in front of us and I flinched.

'Relax doc, it's probably just a stray round,' said James, 'If they were aiming for us we'd be dead by now; they're quite accurate when they want to be.'

'Accurate, I've heard that somewhere,' I said.

We reached the gate; two cars pulled up at once and two burly men hurried forward.

'We got the message,' they said, 'Are you the doctor?'

By this time, interrogations by secret organizations had ceased to terrify me.

'No,' I said, 'The name's Bond; James Bond. We need to get this kid to the hospital right now. Both of you, take him by the shoulders; gently, gently.'

The nearest car was a large jeep and there was plenty of room in the back. Whatever burst of energy and lucidity James had displayed on the hill was now well spent, and he slumped down in the seat, head lolling, eyes vacant, drool glistening at the side of his mouth.

'Straight to hospital, get someone to phone ahead and tell them, fractured femur, significant blood loss …' I began, then I looked back.

I saw a small figure retreating backwards across the field, gunfire still rattling in the air. As I watched he staggered, fell, struggled to get up, fell again, then finally lay still; it almost looked part of a Charlie Chaplin comedy routine, without the gouts of blood, red wouldn't have shown up properly in the old black and white movies. Another martyr for old Ireland, I thought.

'Go ahead without me,' I told them, 'We're going to need another bloody song.'

I ran back through the gate and across the field.

Anton was face-up, a deep gash across his temple

Another shot rang out, and I looked down in puzzlement, feeling a pain in my chest; a red blotch appeared on my shirt.

I felt weak and sagged to my knees.

'Anton …' I tried to speak; blood bubbled from my lips and I slumped to the ground.

'Looks like we're both martyrs,' whispered Anton as darkness fell.

The value of life

BMJ 12 September 1998

A few weeks ago, I visited W B Yeats's grave and sat awhile in thought; no towers of adamant nor rings of steel, just a simple stone monument with the words, 'Cast a cold eye/ On life, on death/Horseman pass by.'

A few hours later and a few miles south, I was in a bar on the Atlantic coast, drinking a pint of the blackest porter, eating crab claws fresh from the sea and soaking in garlic butter, and hammering away at my guitar in an impromptu folk music session. Pausing to check that the kids were still alive (exposure to bitter north west gales and twelve-foot waves being an essential ingredient of the magic of childhood) I fell into conversation with a local, who, on the ubiquitous subject of famous literary graves, told me proudly that Dr Oliver St John Gogarty was buried nearby.

Oliver St John Gogarty was unflatteringly immortalised as Buck Mulligan in James Joyce's *Ulysses*, but he was a substantial literary figure in his own right, and like most of us substantial literary figures he needed the day job to make a buck; further evidence of how the vocations of medicine and literature constitute a fecund union. It was he who performed the autopsy on Michael Collins, Ireland's lost leader, assassinated at Beal na Blath in 1922. Gogarty died in America, and his body was flown home in a lead lined coffin. He was buried with all honours a nation could bestow, in a graveyard overlooking the ocean, and a few weeks later the natives dug him up and sold the lead.

In the middle of this happiness, as if from another universe, comes news of the car bomb in Omagh. All day a steadily mounting death toll; it has reached 28, but the unborn twins were 36 weeks' gestation and surely warrant to be counted among the dead. If you were to bake a cake of sorrow the ingredients could not have been more carefully chosen: the unborn twins; the unknowing foreign students; the little children; the three generations of one family—all wiped out in an instant. But paradoxically the bomb was indiscriminate; nationalist, unionist, old, young, shopkeeper, shopper.

I've been close to several bombs, and it's the sounds I remember most, a dread pattern; the deafening blast, then the stunned silence, as if in an instant the damage is being measured, and then the cries, of two distinct kinds, the same, yet unmistakably different: cries due to injury and pain, and keening due to sorrow and loss and hearts broken in the blink of an eye.

There is a strong sense that this tragedy is the last, shuddering spasm of the Troubles, that no more can be tolerated; no more grief, the peace process must work. It is sickening that this act was performed with the noble aspiration of a united Ireland.

'To be greatly and effectively wicked,' as C S Lewis observed, 'a man needs some virtue.'

The real war against terrorism

BMJ 6 May 2004

My practice is only a stone's throw (medium sized stone, choose one with a rough texture for an easy grip, use an overhand cast—you learn about these things growing up in Ulster) from the border with the Republic of Ireland,

and was particularly hard hit by the Troubles. Deprivation, unemployment, and despair were a lethal cocktail, and after seeing so many young lives wrecked, I am a confirmed pacifist. Violence begets violence, and perceived injustice and repression is the best recruiting programme any paramilitary organisation could desire.

I know too little about the Iraq war for my opinion to be worth anything; it doesn't help that I don't believe anything I read any more. I have learnt from my experience in Ulster that anyone close enough to the situation to really know what's going on is too close to be objective, while anyone distant enough to be objective is also too distant to really know what's going on. An informed yet objective opinion is rare, and when it does appear, is impossible to pick out against all the other plausibly argued but unbalanced opinions.

Saddam was obviously not a benevolent ruler, and just because there are so many other tyrannical regimes in the world doesn't mean it wasn't right to terminate this one. But prosperous godfathers were a feature of the Troubles in Ireland as well, and, as usual, in Iraq those who pulled the first trigger were sitting safely back in the White House.

Hypothetically the man who declares war should be the first one over the top. Dealing death is much more antiseptic when you are thousands of miles away; you don't actually understand what it is you do, you don't see a young man's head exploding, you don't smell burnt flesh, you don't comprehend the thousands of individual tragedies.

I may know little about Iraq, but practising medicine in Ulster has given me some hard-earned insight into the cause and cure of terrorism; I've seen too many of those individual tragedies at painfully close quarters.

The only true war on terror will be a war on poverty, ignorance, and injustice. It will be a long war, and it won't be a war that will make viewer-friendly headlines on CNN, but it is the only war which will have any chance of success.

Be alert

BMJ 4 August 2005

The more things change, the more they stay the same—cynical old men suckering gullible and vulnerable young men into doing their dirty work for them. You've just experienced it in London, I saw it for years in Northern Ireland.

You'll get used to it. More visible security, regular searches, frequent false alarms, delays on trains and buses—all these things will gradually soften like music into the background. Life has to go on, the anxiety will fade as you adjust to a different dynamic, you'll go back to talking about football and the weather, and patients will still want antibiotics for colds and sore throats even as the sirens wail. Humans aren't genetically designed for absolute tranquillity, and a bit of uncertainty is probably good for us.

Statistically the chances of being involved are slight. During the Troubles about 3000 people were killed, and in that same period the death toll on the roads was over 6000. But the increased threat does make you more alert to small things, a little bit more cautious and thoughtful.

I was driving to a house call when I noticed a cardboard box at the side of the road. I stopped the car and sat for a while, pondering. It was just a cardboard box on a small country road, almost certainly just a piece of stray litter;

no wires, no traditional whiff of cordite, no gunfire, no sign of any 'insurgents,' nothing at all suspicious.

I got out of the car at a prudent distance and looked sternly at the box; I consider myself an alpha male. It looked back at me, unblinking. Observing the conventions, it exuded a faint air of menace: 'You're alive, you're dead,' it seemed to be saying, 'it really doesn't matter to me.' For a long moment neither of us moved.

Then I turned around and made a detour which cost me 10 miles; fortune may favour the brave, but the devil hates a coward.

Death or glory?

BMJ 13 August 1994

Crossmaglen has a legendary, if infamous, name and people shudder when they hear where I practise. But, in truth, it is a very pleasant place to work; they are good people, and you can get used to anything, even helicopters flying overhead all day; and working in a place where there is no police presence does add an extra interest to our duties. Occasionally, however, even this professional equanimity can be disturbed.

This call came just after midnight. A mortar had been fired at the security base that afternoon and the van used to launch the mortar had been booby trapped, exploding when brought to the base. I'd heard the bang, and as usual, was mentally estimating how far away it was, and how large.

As I pulled up my conspicuously white car under the arc lights outside the base, I could hear shots. I confess with no modesty that I was more irritated than scared; when you're a doctor, you're a doctor, and you gotta do these things, don't you?

I unloaded my cumbersome and inappropriately fluorescent emergency bags and tottered across the road. As I approached the door of the base it opened, and a squad of troops came running out and dived to the ground in the verges.

I couldn't help but notice how they were all wearing helmets, khaki camouflage, and bulletproof vests, while I was staggering around in the middle of the road, feeling like I should have a big target painted on my chest or be wearing a teeshirt, 'I am an idiot, please shoot me.' So it was with a fatal satisfaction beyond fear that I saw the ground at my feet being scuffed up.

They say you don't hear the shot that hits you; well, you don't hear the ones that make you dance either. The human mind has many powerful denial mechanisms; my life was in danger, and I was thinking that if I was in England I'd be getting a bloody medal for this; meeting the Queen, like, and her saying, 'And what do you do?'

Me: I am a GP in Crossmaglen, ma'am.

Queen: How interesting.

Me: Yes, ma'am, it's quite a lark.

Duke: Here is your medal, my brave lad.

Me: Thanks, but medals don't go down well where I come from.

Red Queen: Off with his head!

Carrollian whimsy is a potent defence against our existentialist fears. I also realised that these were stray bullets, presenting as I did an unmissable target. So I survived to tell this tale.

Afterwards I reflected what good experience this would have been for a student or trainee, but these are rare birds in an area like ours; at least they could have held up the white flag for me. I also considered submitting the case report to the Journal of General Practice, but decided against it, reckoning that it would be turned down because I had no control group and my series was not statistically significant.

Just part of the rich tapestry that is general practice, I guess.

Footnote; in 1994 the British Medical Journal had a competition for a new columnist and this was my winning entry. It was lucky break and kick-started my writing career. Obviously, the shock value of the column was crucial, the realisation that a family doctor in the UK could be doing this kind of stuff.

Chapter 11

The NHS

The NHS is a solemn contract we make together: even if you are sick, or vulnerable, you won't be left behind. Some of us may be lucky and never cost a penny, others unlucky and require a lot of expensive care; over the millions of us that make the contract, it evens out. No-one gets left behind, though it may be a while before they are picked up. We all share the comfort of the security blanket.

There's no luxury, it's the Ryanair health service with no frills - it aims to give you what you need, rather than what you want. We take it for granted, and we won't miss it till it's gone. To paraphrase Winston Churchill, 'The NHS may not be a good system of healthcare, except when you compare it with all the rest.'

Private medicine's real manifesto

BMJ 1 July 2013

Historians may one day look back and say that there was a time, in the 20th century, when people actually gave a fuck about each other. That once the world was more than just a jungle— a pasture of savage beasts, of monsters rising on all sides to smite us, where the strong prosper and the weak are devoured.

But that time is passing, as our health minister perfects the trick of throwing up his hands in horror while simultaneously washing them, like a little Tory Pontius Pilate. And as the NHS is slowly eroded, private medicine is blossoming. It even has a conference now: Private Practice 2013 is *'for clinicians looking to launch or expand their private practice'* and who *'want to start a private practice and offer a higher quality service.'* So it's timely to present the real manifesto for private medicine.

- 1) Always remember that you are a client, not a patient. Your main purpose is for us to generate income. Our doctors will be professional, I'm sure, but if you do happen to get better, that's just a bonus.

- 2) Health is a commodity, disease the product line, and doctors the sales force. We'll obfuscate with weasel words like 'providing a better service,' but remember point 1.

- 3) We do things to you; that's what we do. There is money in procedures. Sitting you in a bed and watching you for a few days is not a big earner. Masterly inactivity will not launch us into the million dollar club.

- 4) Old, chronically ill, or mentally ill people are unsuitable for our services.

- 5) Private health screens are the whores of medicine. They make even us a bit ashamed.

- 6) 'Robes and furred gowns hide all / Plate sin with gold, / And the strong lance of justice hurtless breaks.' We disguise our mendacity with a veneer of luxury. The waiting room has carpet and ferns, and you won't have to share it with the riff raff.

- 7) When I was a young lad I briefly worked in private practice, and a senior colleague told me, 'Take the money off them when the tears are in their eyes.'

- Of course, if the worst happens and you get really sick (or unprofitable) you will be turfed back to the NHS. Looking after sick people: that's what the NHS is for, isn't it?

Dragons' Den

GP 12 November 2008

The dragons looked as smug and self-satisfied as ever, even though studies have proved that wealthy people are 25 per cent unhappier than the rest of us - actually not true, but something to hold on to. The whole thing was rather degrading, but desperate times call for desperate measures and the NHS is seriously short of cash.

'My proposal is quite simple; that we look after sick people, and try to make them better,' I began.

'And how much can we charge them?' interrupted a particularly oily dragon; they were all oily, it was just a matter of degree.

'I don't think you quite understand,' I explained, 'we won't be charging them anything; no luxuries, but all healthcare will be free.'

'So what are your projected profits going to be?' was the next question.

'There will be no profits,' I repeated, grovelling and cringing in an attempt to fit in. 'We aren't looking for profits.'

'There must be a catch; you tie them into a deal when they are sick and vulnerable, bamboozle them with jargon, flog them insurance or something, and then put the arm into them later on, is that it?'

'No,' I said, 'we are not trying to swindle them out of their life-savings, this is not the USA. We are just trying to make sick people better; it's not complicated.'

'So what's in it for us?'

'How about the satisfaction of doing something good and noble instead of being a greedy capitalist pig?'

'No, seriously,' said Oily, unimpressed.

'At least they must be pretty grateful for all this free stuff,' greased a fat lady dragon.

'Well, no,' I admitted, 'gratitude is not a plant that thrives in the NHS, unlike complaints.'

'Complaints?' objected a dragon, spitting at a passing toady. 'All this free care and they are allowed to complain?'

'And there are patient satisfaction surveys as well,' I explained, realising that more and more this was not sounding like an attractive business proposal.

'That's poor people for you, wanting something for nothing,' said a dragon with a long flowing perm. 'There's no money in this, let's go back to the USA.'

'Or stick with complementary medicine,' said another.

Selling fear? First make people scared

GP 28 March 2018

A member of my family had surgery last year. The surgeon was from Pakistan, the anaesthetist from Spain, the recovery nurse from Italy, the ward nurse from the Philippines, the SHO from the UK. An international array of talents and skills, this kind of global cooperation is what makes the NHS the precious institution that it is, people from all over the world working together to make our patients better. Foreigners are not enemies, not antagonists, not people to be feared. Foreigners and refugees didn't cause the banking crisis which led to the years of austerity; it was the banks, remember?

How far we have fallen since the London Olympics; the energy, the dynamism and the formidable organisation throughout the fortnight, the creativity and self-confidence of the opening and closing ceremonies, all underlining London's place as one of the centres of the world.

But the dream is shattered, and we have become inward-looking and fearful and divided and diminished. We used to aspire to intelligence, now we ridicule 'experts'. As Isaac Asimov said: 'Anti-intellectualism has been a constant thread winding its way through our political and cultural life, nurtured by the false notion that democracy means that 'my ignorance is just as good as your knowledge.'

That Donald Trump became president of the USA was a bewildering spectacle from this side of the world. In any other civilised country, a presidential candidate who mocked a disabled person would have been immediately disqualified; perhaps this is what is meant by American Exceptionalism? But his election has to be put in the context of Brexit and that £500 cajillion for the NHS canard.

Where do you hide a leaf? In a forest. Where do you hide a lie? In a Forest of Lies.

The campaigns of poorly-concealed envy and mistrust and egotism had a painful logic; when you sell sausages you don't wait for people to want sausages, you go out and make them hungry. When you want to appeal to intolerance and bigotry, you make people feel afraid and victimised.

When you want to sell fear, you go out and make people scared.

The subtle art of dementia screening

GP 9 May 2014

Joe may be officially retired, but, admirably, he keeps himself active, dry-gulching farmers and smuggling rare and irreplaceable wild orchids. So when I saw his multi-purpose HiAce van outside the house, I seized the opportunity.

I haven't been a GP for the past 20 years without learning an embarrassing secret or two, so I used the Secret Knock of the Royal Horticultural Society.

Joe, ever suspicious of fellow orchid-traffickers (they are known for their ruthlessness, which is why the Colombian cartels have never cracked the market), opened the door an inch.

When he saw me, he tried to slam it, but too late; I had my foot in the door - a foot of iron, bolstered by a dread purpose.

'I am here, Joe,' I said solemnly, with just a hint of a threat, accidentally/deliberately kicking over an expensive flowerpot, 'to screen you for dementia.'

'Honestly, doc, I'm fine, I'm feeling great,' he protested, doing a little twerk to emphasise his animal vitality, but he had a guilty look on his face. Admittedly, Joe always has a guilty look on his face, because he is always guilty of something.

'You may think you are well, Joe,' I said, 'but that's because we haven't investigated you enough yet.'

Apparently early diagnosis of dementia is now desirable, despite the real priority being support systems for the patients we've already diagnosed.

As Dr Martin Brunet argued recently in the BMJ: 'Dementia is big business, and there are many vested interests that stand to benefit from a rise in the number of diagnoses. Currently the use of diagnosis target rates is proving to be a highly successful strategy for politicians and industry.'

Asking patients the queen's name has become redundant, because they can Google it on their smartphones, so I prefer open questions.

'What is your favourite colour?' I asked.

'Red?' he said, cracking under the strain. 'No, wait, it's blue, I meant blue!'

'Too late,' I said, coldly.

Warning! Humans working in the NHS

GP 3 March 2014

'It is always the best policy to speak the truth,' said Jerome K Jerome, who then added an important qualification - 'Unless, of course, you are an exceptionally good liar.'

So we all owe a debt of gratitude to leading surgeon Professor J Meirion Thomas; his unpalatable truth is that 'the gender imbalance is already having a negative effect on the NHS'.

Most female doctors, he explained, end up working part-time - usually in general practice. They tend to avoid the more demanding specialties, which require greater commitment, and look for a better work/life balance.

Doctors also tend to marry within their own socio-economic group and, he observes, in many cases, the wife is the secondary earner, which further encourages less demanding part-time work. Not only lazy bitches, you see, but lazy and snobby bitches as well.

The professor also pointed out that as: 'GPs tend to work in small group practices, there is a danger these can become backwaters, isolated from the nourishing influences of hospital medicine.' The obvious solution, which he probably omitted for brevity, is for everybody to live close to a hospital.

General practice, he concluded, is organised for the convenience of doctors - particularly female GPs - not their patients. As you might expect, there was fierce condemnation of the professor's remarks from the usual suspects, all aflame with righteous outrage; we can't handle the truth.

In reality, the professor's honesty didn't go far enough. I can reveal that there are also men working in the NHS. Let's be honest, men are pigs; I'm one, so I should know. Shallow, venal creatures, exhibiting all the vices, except perhaps greed, which requires a bit of energy.

How the NHS continues to function with such a large percentage of men and women in the workforce is a mystery. The truth is, you can get a lot done when you don't have, you know, a life.

Sometimes I think I care too much

GP 5 July 2013

'I've an awful sore throat,' said Joe, 'and I've been fighting it all week.'

There followed an expectant silence, while Joe waited for the traditional sarcastic response: 'Fighting it all week? Want a medal?'

But I've changed.

'You've been fighting it all week, all alone in the dark watches of the night,' I said, my voice heavy with emotion, my lower lip quivering. 'You brave soul, what torment you have endured.'

I took out a lavender-scented kerchief and wiped away a tear.

'My friend, this is not a battle you have to face alone.' I stood up and advanced, as Joe shrank back in his chair. 'What about a hug?' I said

Horrified as he was, Joe is nothing if not game, and we shared a manly if uncomfortable hug.

Yes, I've changed, but why have I changed? Events, dear boy, events; on the surface I may seem profound and sympathetic, but deep down I'm superficial and manipulative.

Incredibly, compassion is now to be evaluated, and not as you might think, as a QOF point along with lust and sloth. According to Professor Nigel Sparrow of the CQC, the CQC intends to evaluate the 'less easily measured aspects of general practice' and 'things to do with care, compassion and values'.

Professor Sparrow said: 'When I used to visit practices for training practice accreditation, I used to spend a few minutes sitting in the waiting room and those few minutes were extraordinarily valuable. It gives you a general impression of how caring and compassionate those staff are.'

Well, I have nothing to hide; the professor is welcome to squat in our waiting room anytime, magazines only 10 years old and one-armed bandits to keep our gambling addicts quiet. Visit the toilets as well, I suggest, one place where there are no secrets and men tell each other the truth.

Joe gently disengaged himself from the hug.

'Never knew you were so compassionate, doc,' he said.

'You're still not getting any antibiotics,' I sobbed.

Taking time to cut through the niceties

GP 4 July 2012

'Thanks, doc,' said Joe, pocketing his protection money and getting up to leave.

'Hold your horses,' I said. 'It has been ordained by the NHS that GP consultations should last 50% longer.'

'Really?' said Joe, fascinated by the concept that I wanted him to stay a bit longer, he being well aware that when I tell him to 'take care' I actually mean 'take off'.

'Which gives you,' I said, making a rapid calculation, 'another 30 seconds.'

'OK,' said Joe, always happy to co-operate.

We sat twiddling our thumbs in silence; I'm happy with silence, I could listen to it all day, especially during surgery hours. But Joe was less serene.

'This is nice,' he said, uncomfortably.

By this time in a Zen-like trance, I did not respond, and Joe felt something further was needed.

'Maybe you could give me some lifestyle advice,' he said.

Irritated by having to return prematurely to planet Earth, I was a bit more brusque than usual.

'No problem,' I said. 'You're too fat.'

Joe was discommoded by my bluntness.

'That's not very nice, doctor,' he said, 'I thought doctors were supposed to be more supportive, less judgmental.' 'Niceness doesn't enter into it,' I said, 'To paraphrase W.B. Yeats, I do not tread softly for fear of treading on your dreams. It's my duty to tell it like it is; a dirty job, but somebody's gotta do it.'

'But shouldn't you break it to me gently,' said Joe, 'Maybe I have a slow metabolism, or big bones or something.'

This, I had to admit, was a good point.

'Big bones, big belly, big arse, you have the complete collection,' I agreed.

'You're much too negative,' he said. 'I could do with a bit of positive thinking.'

'I'm your doctor, not your buddy,' I said, drawing a little Venn diagram to demonstrate this dictum in a mathematical format; a circle labelled doctor and a circle labelled patient with a big space, a metaphorical desk, in between them.

'So I'm fat,' said Joe. 'What should I do about it?'

'Your time is up,' I said. 'Take care.'

Appraisal (Part 1)

GP Feb 11 2010

'You disgust me,' he said, 'you and your fancy shirts and your fast women and your big shiny car. Well, let me tell you, joy-boy, it cuts no ice with me.'

Some of this was quite flattering, so I didn't protest.

276

'I'd like to leap over this desk,' he went on, 'rip out your stinking guts and wrap them round your neck.'

The appraisal was not going well. We had gotten off to a bad start – he hadn't been impressed by the old The Dog Ate My Portfolio excuse.

I was a bit taken aback by this degree of aggression, wistfully remembering a kinder gentler time, when appraisal was more chummy and congenial, something to look forward to, a comfortable fireside chat between colleagues, a friendly exchange of views over tea and freshly-baked scones.

And if my appraiser was a child of the 60s, we'd reminisce fondly of Woodstock and 'sticking it to the man' and sex and drugs and rock'n'roll and how we were going to change the world and 'give peace a chance', maybe even get our old kaftans out, get naked for a while, light up a joss stick or two, check out the vibe, hold hands, wear flowers in our hair and sing a few verses of Kumbaya, until eventually the receptionist would interrupt and be only mildly surprised to find us frothing at the mouth.

I considered my response; common sense might have dictated a soothing tone at this point, but we GPs are a maverick, feisty bunch, and we don't kowtow lightly to authority, nor react kindly to coercion.

The French have a phrase – *la trahison des clercs*; i.e. the treachery of the intellectuals, for those who are aware of abuses but fail to confront them. Perhaps this was the moment to make a stand, to rage against the machine, to demand that appraisal be reckoned a constructive rather than a punitive process.

I chose the soothing tone; a cop-out, you might think, but don't shoot me, after all these years in general practice apathy is the only emotion I keep handy.

'Hey,' I said, in the soothing (and patronising) tone I use for counselling, which I also know to be particularly aggravating, 'Why so hostile? You're OK, I'm OK.'

In a fury, he flung my PDP at me and stormed out. A single page tore loose and floated slowly to the floor, like a little teardrop, I mused.

There is a possibly apocryphal, yet potentially enlightening story from Ceausescu's Romania. An associate producer at Romanian TV suggested it would be a good idea to show a nightly 10-minute review of the dictator's activities. The next toady up the pecking order suggested 10 minutes wasn't enough, it had to be 30 minutes, and so on and on, until the people had to endure three hours on the leader's activities every night.

Ideas have momentum and stopping them is like jumping in front of a train. Assessing doctors' performance is obviously a Good Idea, isn't it? Who could reasonably object? But this idea midwifed the sulky child of appraisal, which has in turn matured into the evil goblin of revalidation.

There are vested interests thriving here and the goblin has become like a living being; the original remit, to ensure doctors practise to an acceptable standard, has been lost, and its real mission now is to grow, extend its influence, employ more lackeys, and bump up the salaries and pensions of its senior management. This labyrinthine bureaucracy will cost, apparently, more than £1bn.

But, I hear you say, without revalidation or appraisal, how would we track down the massive problem of underperforming doctors? Actually, it's not massive, it's

278

less than 1% of doctors, and I have a solution, which is cheaper and more fun; we should employ counter-insurgency techniques and simply grass them up.

I'd have no problem informing on any of my colleagues, in the interests of the greater good; provided, of course, that the phone-line was completely confidential.

I wouldn't want any unpleasantness.

Appraisal (part deux)

GP June 4 2018

It is commonly understood that there are two types of appraiser. Most are permanently malcontent, their disposition suggesting a recent series of disappointing bowel movements. The initial conversation may be polite, yet beneath the veneer of civility lurks only ugly suspicion; handshakes above the table and loaded guns below.

But there is another type, the type of appraiser who really wants to be your friend, and would pass you even if your portfolio was accidentally on purpose stained with insalubrious body fluids. In a Kafkaesque indulgence I shall call the appraiser K.

K peered suspiciously at the stains.

'It's just coffee,' I said reassuringly.

'Might have spilt some, I was so nervous about this appraisal, you know,' I explained, yawning hugely, my traitorous body making a liar out of me.

'And your reflective learning?' K asked.

I passed over a few tatty sheets.

'Been working on this all year,' I lied again (my years in general practice have made me quite accomplished at dissimulation). 'Trying to comprehend the importance of sympathy; did I say sympathy? I meant empathy, of course, sympathy is second rate stuff; empathy is the cat's pyjamas.'

'This is very…unusual,' said K, looking over it. 'There is this bit… "Yeah, when you walk in the Valley of Shadow of Death, I'll be right behind you." What does that mean?'

'It means when my patient is walking though the Valley of Shadow of Death, I'll be right behind them,' I explained helpfully. 'It's safer that way; if an alien suddenly bursts out of their chest, I won't be in the firing line.'

There was a long silence as K struggled with the dissonant genres.

'And this,' K continued, '"To take arms against a sea of patients, And by opposing end them". ' That sounds curiously familiar to me.

'And "Patients are like a box of chocolates, you never know what you're going to get till you open them up".'

I wondered if K was cottoning on to my cunning plan, How to Make Reflective Learning Painless by copying a bunch of one-liners from *The Big Book of Quotations*. But there remains medicine's Golden Rule; if you can't baffle them with brilliance, boggle them with bullshit.

'I was interweaving my literary influences with my own experience,' I said, extemporising i.e. lying.

'Ah, now I understand,' said K.

'Thanks,' I said. 'That's so empathetic of you.'

Chapter 12

House calls

Some birds aren't meant to be caged; their plumage is just too bright. Which is why every family doctor loves the house-call; to escape the unbearable ennui of our desk-bound prison, to flap our wings and fly, to drive free and clear along dappled leaf-strewn country roads, to run naked across the fields (if it's not raining and the cows aren't aggressive).

But it's not always as pleasant as it sounds......

A bloody mess at the garden party...

GP 7 April 2011

It was a blissful, halcyon summer's day; sun shining, blue skies, birds singing, bees humming and horny goats and rabbits everywhere. So an emergency house call to a garden party seemed quite appropriate.

As it was an emergency, and as I am sometimes A Good Doctor, I dropped everything (leaving behind the queue of sick certs and passport applications, with a heavy heart, of course) and dashed to the house immediately, stopping only to pick up a straw boater, a striped blazer, a picnic of smoked salmon, cucumber and brown bread, a bottle of Pimm's, and to hire a couple of toadies; 20 years in general practice has taught me the importance of always having the right equipment. *Cum stramenta catherise parare omittat plasticae manus ungloved* (fail to prepare, prepare to catheterise with a plastic straw and ungloved hands).

The scene was idyllic; the gentle chatter of effete society, *In a Monastery Garden* playing in the background on an old gramophone, the far-away drone of a small airplane, the tinkle of champagne flutes, the murmurous haunt of flies on summer eves. A good war to thin out the working class and everything would have been almost perfect, marred only by the bloody mess that used to be Sebastian. Due to a fatal combination of high spirits and low IQ, he had impaled himself on a croquet mallet, apparently an occupational hazard among public schoolboys..

Despite the repulsive spectacle Sebastian had become, the croquet game was continuing with a defiant serenity.

'I say, old boy', said a splendid old gentleman with a moustache which had an uncanny (though no doubt accidental) similarity to a diagram of the uterus and fallopian tubes (the clinician in me never sleeps), 'Would you mind shifting that blood clot? It's interfering with my backswing.'

That's the spirit that made the British Empire great, I thought.

A fragrant young lady fainted, but carefully, so as not to get her dress dirty.

'Oh, my darling Priscilla', said the dowager. 'Quick, doctor, do something, and someone get me another gin, and this time leave the bottle.'

After 20 years in general practice I've learnt to handle even the most unusual clinical situations.

'Gosh, Priscilla', I said, 'you've fainted on a slug.'

The cure was instantaneous.

Quaint or what?

BMJ 15 July 2000

The hills are beautiful at this time of the year; the verdant meadows tranquil but for the racket of bumblebees frenziedly rogering the butterflies among the dandelions and the Great God Pan making lewd suggestions to the wood nymphs; whin bushes golden and so lush with spines that if you threw in a herbalist she would squeal for weeks; snow white lily-of-the-valley coating the glen-sides like talcum powder down the natal cleft of a big fat man, as Wordsworth might have said if he had had medical training.

And the people; slow, sullen, and yet dull, we are so rural that cows are considered effete, stylised, and possibly homosexual, and the only thing we milk is the social security system. We are unsentimental about nature; we can't eat the scenery, we say, though judging from our dental appearance, some of us have tried, so we augment our incomes by smuggling and by blackmailing small furry animals.

Hunt saboteurs find us unsympathetic, although we dislike fat upper-class bastards on horseback just as much as they do; if a fox could eat you, we assure them, it would, and it wouldn't care if it had to hunt you bare-arsed across the hills to do it. As for tree huggers, the day a tree hugs you back, you'll be sorry. According to a local folk-song, French kiss an oak tree and you end up with a mouthful of gloopy sap.

We are shy and terse, and we follow the Bible's teaching: 'Never let your left hand know what your right hand is doing,' it advises, to which I add, especially when it involves bodily organs. One of the joys of visiting other countries is engaging in discourse with the locals and learning about their culture, so tourists here are completely fucked.

The police enjoy all the esteem of a dead goat, and a doctor's life accordingly becomes more diverting.

'My brother's cut himself, I want you to come out and stitch him up.'

I explained that such a brutal injury would need to attend the surgery.

'There's no one for to drive him.'

I remained firm, and eventually the real reason emerged.

'We can't bring him in, he's threatening us with a knife.'

Footnote; Someone wasn't too pleased with this article, and wrote to the BMJ thus;

One for the gutter

Dear Editor,

I read with mounting incredulity the disjointed and offensive article on page 185 of this week's BMJ under the title of 'Soundings'. I had to turn to the front of the journal to confirm that I was actually reading the BMJ. I then considered whether there was an erudite message that I had missed; something on a higher plain with hidden implication. After reading it again I reverted to my original interpretation that the piece was more suitable for the lowest form of gutter press. I am all in favour of freedom of expression but I would expect that a publication such as the BMJ would pride itself on maintaining a reasonably professional standard in relation to its contents. To be charitable, I concede that living in 'Bandit Country' may have a deleterious effect on the intellect.

But I was not without support, as the next letter showed;

Dear Editor,

Re: One for the gutter

As a rural resident, but not in 'Bandit country', I know just what Liam Farrell is getting at. I hope he won't be put off by intemperate and ill considered responses (like this one!) but will continue to delight and entertain with his pieces.

A winter's tale; are you the fucking doctor?

BMJ   3 January 2008

Global warming is no picnic for general practitioners; it has irrevocably altered the aesthetic of wintertime home visits, a cherished part of general practice since the day Asclepius first said, 'Art thou sure thou can't come in to the surgery?'

Gone forever are the days of snow-covered hills, frost coldly rimming the meadows, rich beds and bright fires and hot whiskeys, big mugs of tea and freshly baked scones, what Ratty and his little furry life-partner, before coming out of the closet, (and boy, was that a shock for the Woodland Community, though they're cool with it now) would have called midwinter's homely comforts. House calls then were a wonderland, like being in a Disney movie starring Dr Finlay and James Herriot, and getting jiggy with Julie Andrews by the final credits.

But now all is utterly changed; it's just mud and misery from October to April.

So instead of tap-dancing through the farmyard on a crisp magical white carpet of freshly fallen snow, I was in muck to the knees, and it wasn't just non-organic muck; the mandatory herd of cows had added their enthusiasm to the mix, the result being a cocktail of steaming malodorous ordure that would have given even the mighty Hercules pause for thought; 'Not more bloody cows,' he'd have said, 'The Augean Stables were bad enough, give me the Nemean Lion any day.'

I squelched to the door.

'Now is the winter of our discontent made summer by this glorious . . . ' I began, as a bit of scholarship always goes down well with our stout yeomanry, but I was interrupted; the usual warm Irish welcome had become, with bitter irony, much colder.

'Are you the fucking doctor?' I was asked.

I explained carefully, not wishing any misunderstanding, that I was just the ordinary doctor; to be a fucking doctor required a further qualification, many years of arduous postgraduate study at Cambridge University culminating in a demanding final examination in which the most critical element was, for obvious reasons, the oral, after which you were awarded a magnificent diploma and a jar of anti-fungal cream.

Patient confidentiality forbids me describing the consultation which followed; suffice to say it was short and concluded with a prescription for antibiotics, just to show How Much I Care.

Global warming or not, some things never change.

The Unforgettable Dr Farrell

BMJ 25 August 2009

'You're a marvellous doctor,' she said. I shuffled my feet uneasily. We Irish are a modest race, but this is a veneer only, and 'You're a marvellous doctor' was, I felt, quite inadequate to describe the wonder that is me; I wanted a parade, a brass band, Mickey Mouse, stars climbing the dew-dropping sky just to light my passing feet, Angelina Jolie weeping by the phone the next day because I hadn't called her.

'And little Johnny thinks you're wonderful,' she said.

'Children have a way of seeing things clearly, don't you think?' I allowed.

'Just one thing,' she said, 'that outfit may scare him. He's very sensitive.'

The swine flu protective gear was a bit intimidating, I had to agree, as though I had been driving through plutonium.

'So,' she continued, 'if you could take it off and then come to the window where Johnny can see you put it on again he'll know it's dear old Dr Farrell, not some monster fixing to burst out of his stomach. In retrospect, I probably shouldn't have let him watch *Alien*.'

The wonderful and so easily manipulated Dr Farrell could hardly refuse such a request, and I began to disrobe. It had been a serene summer's day, but a capricious little squall displayed precise timing. My cap flew off into a nearby leylandii; a flock of pigeons exploded out, liquidly venting their outrage. One apron cord got tangled in an overhead power cable, there was a fizzing noise and my hair caught fire; a passing eucalyptus went up like a torch.

The bib flapped over my face as the other apron cord sneakily wrapped itself round my legs. Blinded, dazed, in agonising pain, and stinking of guano, I blundered across the garden, smashing headlong into the bird table, which had been thoughtfully stocked that very morning.

287

A cascade of seeds, nuts, and mealworms rained down upon me, followed by a second wave of ravenous tits, wrens, chaffinches, and a crazed and disoriented woodpecker (there are no woodpeckers in Ireland, apparently).

By this time the whole neighbourhood had gathered in to see what I'd do next; an ice cream van, sensing a commercial opportunity, tinkled a merry tune.

Fortunately, a torrential shower intervened, dousing the flames. I discarded the pathetic remnants of the protective suit and went in to examine Johnny.

'You'll be fine,' I told him.

'Who are you?' he replied.

Footnote; Remember when swine flu was the new black?

Footnote 2; There are now woodpeckers in Ireland.

Adventures of a little black bag

GP 15 May 2015

My little black bag, my faithful companion for more than 20 years. Black fading to a dignified grey, the bouquet of old leather, a thousand memories.

Open it up and it's like the Tardis, defying the space-time continuum, much bigger on the inside. Like a part of me, I can find what I want without looking, just by rummaging around, ignoring the risk of being stabbed by an errant scalpel.

Stethoscope, sphyg, ophthalmoscope (for theatrical purposes), thermometer, torch, prescription pad, these are but the bare bones; my bag is multipurpose.

If you get hungry while warding off the forces of darkness, you can have a snack; there's always a half-eaten sandwich somewhere in the depths, or a few ancient toffees stuck to the lining. And an ersatz tracheostomy kit - an old ball-point pen, in case someone needs an emergency tracheostomy, after which Meg Ryan will sleep with me in gratitude (I've seen this in the movies, so it must be true).

The fancy climate-controlled aluminium gigs are not for me. I prefer vintage, a visible manifestation of our ancient profession's authority. And vintage is heavier, which can come in handy.

The guard dog, apparently half-sheepdog and half-hyena, was in a frenzy, leaping up and snapping at the car door, spattering the window with drool, such was his excitement at the prospect of tasting family doctor flesh.

I'm a lover, not a fighter, but there was a patient waiting with an 'awful' sore throat and my vocation - to cure sometimes, comfort always, be sarcastic whenever possible - would not be denied.

Cometh the hour, cometh the doc; if you can't stand the heat, get out of general practice.

'Say hello to my little friend,' I snarled in my best Al Pacino accent, swinging my trusty black bag like the sword of retribution and bludgeoning the surprised dog into a corner of the barnyard.

'Now the beast cannot harm you,' I declaimed to the world.

I don't know about the patient, but after that visit, I felt much better.

Night thoughts

BMJ 4 February 1995

When the sun goes down, and all good men and women retire to bed after an honest day's toil, terrible things emerge from their sleep and seek soft flesh and hot blood, the true people of the night, vampires, zombies, burglars, embezzlers, muggers, whores and, of course, doctors.

We GPs are solitary creatures; we don't have the comfort of colleagues close by, we toil far away from the comforting breasts of the general hospital, and alone we must face the darkness.

Even in the brightest sunlight, we are aware of the shadows to come, and when the night is falling like blood-dark wine, our heaviest burdens are fear, memories and loneliness. We must march or die, because if we don't do it, who will?

The winter is the season of truth. The land sheds its pretence of Pre-Raphaelite lushness, liberated at last from the imprisoning foliage, like David redeemed by Michaelangelo from his marble tomb, and the ash-keys hang fluttering in the wind on spectral trees which even Spinoza would have found difficult to love. The hilltops are spare and scant enough to set Mussorgsky whistling a tune, and nature takes its clothes off and runs buck naked around the country. The dance goes on, but without the illusory decor. It is a time when we see through to the bare bones of things, and medicine is one of these.

Flaubert (or was it Balzac?—anyway, some French guy) said that no man had really lived till he had walked out of a brothel in the early hours of the morning wanting to throw himself in the river. Now of course I can't comment on that; in rural general practice we don't (usually) have the opportunity to drink the cup of sensuality to its bitterest and most depraved dregs or bury ourselves headlong into the fleshpots of the city, but we do have our own stark truth.

No-one is a real doctor till they've been called out in the wee hours on a freezing winter's night, snow on snow on the ground, to be met at the top of a boreen by a hurricane lamp.

The hurricane lamp is of course utterly theatrical; its purpose is rather to emphasise the severity of the weather and the darkness of the night. It is mandatory that the boreen is impassable by motorised vehicle, but then the house is only 'a good stretch of the legs' away (at least two miles). You realise you have left your wellies behind, look longingly back at your warm car, and for a wild moment consider leaping into the driver's seat and scorching madly away.

Your very heart's desire is to return to your bed's comforting embrace. It's soft and clean and inviting, and there's no-one dying, no blood or vomit. But you don't, do you, because you're a doctor and you gotta do these things; and because it's real medicine, one of our reasons to be.

And who knows what challenge awaits us at the end of the boreen? A drab delivering in a ditch, or some dull opiate being emptied in overdose to the drains; No one should be so sick or vulnerable or remote or alone that a doctor won't be there, reaching out a hand to cure or comfort. And whatever the challenge is, we're the boys and girls who can handle it.

'What hath the night to do with sleep?' said John Milton, and we GPs know just what he was talking about; just call me Dr Acula.

291

To fight the good fight

BMJ 7 October 1995

I have some good news: our profession is still revered and respected, our authority not to be lightly flouted, nor our wishes blithely scouted.

I was called the other night to a domestic scrap, the bait being a possible head injury. The phone message was guttural and almost incoherent, allowing no negotiation: 'You'd better come quick, Doctor, he's real bad,' and in the background I could hear screams, breaking crockery, and the merry clink of bottle on skull, softened almost into music by the distance.

The neighbourhood remains incompatible with any police force, so other authority figures are mandatory at these spontaneous gatherings; either ourselves or the church, or both, although only doctors have a contractual obligation to attend.

When I arrived—suppressing a strange desire to say 'Well, well, what's going on 'ere, then?'—I realised that there were in fact multiple combatants, but the melee parted gratifyingly before me, like the Red Sea before Moses. There was skin and hair flying; blood, sweat, tears, and beers everywhere.

Looking for the injured party, I wandered through the fracas untouched (there are certain conventions which must be observed, even in the fiercest brawl) like Tony Curtis during the custard pie fight in The Great Race. I idly noticed that, despite the almost complete devastation of the rest of the house, the television and video remained miraculously intact, irrefutable evidence that the violence was not mindless, and that there were no psychoses involved. I was accidentally jostled only once.

'Sorry, Doc,' said the offending protagonist.

'No problem, Jemmie,' I reassured him. 'By the way, come and see me in the morning and I'll sew your ear back on.'

I eventually located the nominated casualty. He had that combination of clinical features which GPs and casualty officers all over the world would instantly despatch to Room 101: the smell of alcohol, a scalp bump and abrasion, and the merest suggestion of a hint of loss of consciousness. We know in our heart of hearts that this guy is going to end up in a hospital bed—if not, Sod's law will ordain for him a fractured skull, an extradural haematoma, and a lawsuit.

I knew there was nothing wrong with him, of course, but he was stretchered out in a shroud of martyrdom anyway. His admission would legitimise the injury ('He had to go to hospital!!') and ensure that the feud will continue way beyond our own seed, breed, and generation.

Eventually, and to my total astonishment, by holding up my hands, flapping them in a vague sort of way and shouting 'now, now,' I was able to quell the disturbance, although I then had to listen magisterially to both sides' justification for their misdemeanours. Finally, the owner of the house appeared.

'By the way, Doctor,' he inquired, with exquisite civility, 'who was it that called you out?'

'I believe it was the gentleman next door,' I replied.

'Really? Thank you very much,' he said, excusing himself politely from the company.

I heard his heavy tread going down his own steps, then up his neighbours' steps, the vigorous rap on the door, the door opening, and then, thunderously:

'If you'se ever call the doctor to my house again, I'll be dug out of ye!' followed by a dull but satisfying thud.

Although, of course, I abhor all violence, I allowed myself a discreet smile of approval.

Come dance with me in Ireland

BMJ 25 November 2009

Admit it. You know it. I know it, we all know it: a doctor's most secret and unholy joy is making another doctor look like a klutz. It can be subtle: the almost imperceptible raising of an eyebrow, the almost inaudible indrawing of breath. Or it can be a custard pie in the face.

'Perhaps you could take this call,' said my partner, poker-faced.

I was young, keen as a puppy, and I bounced beamishly out the door. I didn't know the call had come from yet another brow-beaten home help who just couldn't take it anymore and who felt it only fair that the doctor should share in the invective.

The living room was cluttered and forbidding.

'Who are you?' she demanded.

'I'm Dr Farrell,' I said, 'and I just called to see how you . . .'

'Get out, or I'll set the dogs on you.'

I'm easy-going, I don't take offence easily, I presumed the dogs were a metaphor for the John F Kennedy memorial plate whizzing past my head, but a man's gotta know his limitations.

She followed me to the front door.

'Where are you going?' she asked.

'You asked me to leave,' I said.

Her demeanour suddenly changed.

'Arrah, sure don't be listening to me, ochone, ochone, I'm only a poor old woman, I'm not feeling very well.'

Fascinated, and rather moved, I returned to the living room.

'Why don't we check your blood pressure,' I said, usually a safe bet; having your blood pressure taken is like parfait, everyone loves it. But her demeanour had abruptly changed again.

'Get out,' she said, 'before I . . .'

'I know, I know, the dogs,' I said, surmising a fierce territorial instinct centred on the living room and her picture of the Pope slotting a penalty past Stalin; I was learning that enduring insult is just another part of a doctor's shtick. Again she followed.

'Arrah, I'm only a poor old woman, lie me under the greenwood tree …'

The dance went on, in and out, like waves on the sea, a medical hokey-cokey, until eventually I conducted an ersatz consultation on the porch, in the no-man's land between unrestrained fury and overwhelming pathos.

And arriving back at the surgery: 'Hello, I must be going,' sang my partner.

Don't mind the dog

BMJ 19 September 2012

Sitting up in the tree gave me time to reflect. The sick will always be with us, and there are more of them every day, and no matter how much money we pour in, we will always come up short of expectations.

And the sick are not only inconvenient but inconsiderate.

'Don't mind the dog,' I'd been told by the patient over the phone, which ranks right up there in Things GPs Don't Like To Hear. So there I was, cornered like a rat, gratified that animals have different climbing abilities: squirrels are good; cats can manage; rabbits only embarrass themselves trying. Fortunately, big fierce dogs can't.

I tried shouting at the house to attract attention, but only succeeded in startling a nearby vulture. I contemplated leaping from the tree and bolting for the car, but age has withered me; if I was an actor I'd be Brad Pitt's homely chum, the comic relief.

But that which we are, we are; as Nietzsche might have said, 'Cherish your enemies, even big fierce dogs, because they bring out the best in you.' Age has lent me a certain serenity, to make the best of a bad job, to enjoy the small things, like when somebody you dislike gets indicted for a crime and has to spend years in a dank, poorly ventilated penal facility making new and very intimate friends.

If you could get past the slavering monster at the bottom of the tree, the beauty of the Irish countryside was breathtaking, and after relieving myself, as men are wont to do in high places with panoramic views, I whiled away the time by scrawling some obscene graffiti.

I was surprisingly comfortable in the leafy shade, enjoying the cool manure-scented breeze; bumblebees hummed in the foliage, a robin trilled its liquid song, and a butterfly whispered by. If Piglet and Winnie the Pooh had turned up, I wouldn't have been a bit surprised.

But my idyll was all too brief: 'Some there be that shadows kiss / Such have but a shadow's bliss.' The owner appeared, and dragged the dog away and me back into the real world.

'We've been waiting all day for you,' he said accusingly.

The magic of words

BMJ 8 November 2007

In the small yet dull world of the medical columnist, the use of quotations is considered rather jejune and naff. Meant to imply a deep breadth of scholarship—that the writer curls up each night with a good dose of Seneca and a tincture of Molière—what it really means is a well-thumbed Big Book of Quotations, kept in the bathroom, to be consulted at length while the Great Writer strains away.

But an ear for the telling phrase remains an indispensable part of the columnist's armoury, as it saves us thinking them up ourselves.

When I started practice in Crossmaglen there were no road signs, these having been removed by helpful locals to confuse the British Army and other officers of the state; confusing the new general practitioner was just a convenient bonus.

So when I stopped to ask directions from a likely chap, I was wearing my stethoscope prominently, ensuring that I wouldn't be mistaken for the television licence man. He was sitting on a gate, staring aimlessly into the distance, irrefutable evidence of ample local knowledge; one of the immutable laws of the countryside is that the more unworldly you look, the shrewder you are. I was therefore hopeful of lucid advice.

He was glad to be of assistance, though the faraway look never left his eyes.

'You'd be the new doctor then,' he said perspicaciously. 'Continue on for a mile or so, then deny yourself a right;

you'll see a crossroads, keep straight, take the next left at the plastic cow, and the house is right there in front of you, though to actually reach it you'll have to get out of the car and walk in the opposite direction, yeah really, walk away from it, it's counter-intuitive, like the Red Queen in *Through the Looking Glass*, there's a loop in time/space, you cross the Event Horizon, like in *Stargate* . . . '

The directions continued, but I wasn't listening anymore—I had lost him way back; I was enraptured, in a reverie.

Deny yourself a right! Deny yourself a right? What did he mean? What forbidden pleasures, what glorious vista of debauchery and depravity lay down that country road? What was so tempting that I should have to deny it?

I surfaced eventually, gave him a prescription for antibiotics (the traditional gesture of thanks for services rendered), and drove quickly past that right turn, steadfastly looking the other way, resisting the urge to bury myself headlong in the fleshpots. As Oscar Wilde might have said, 'The only way to conquer temptation is to catch an embarrassing disease because of it.'

But sometimes, deep in the night, it haunts me still......

A true hero

GP 8 April 2010

Our bonds run much deeper than mere sex; we are comrades-in-arms, in the trenches together, and if I was asked to take a bullet for them, I would.

District nurses: I couldn't manage without them and their unique combination of knowledge, experience and common sense that continues to survive attempts at hamstringing by ever-increasing red tape.

Occasionally, we do home visits together; tactics are important here. I listen to their advice and then repeat it back in different words so that it looks like it's really my own opinion. If called on for an opinion directly, I will watch her expression closely even as I speak, ready to change tack at any moment and contradict myself if necessary - for example, your ulcer is improving, I don't think we need any more antibiotics (then, observing the merest suggestion of a frown) but it hasn't improved as much as I hoped, so I think we do need antibiotics.

Joe had an extensive and persistent ulcer, and the nurse was busy dressing his leg, while at the head of the bed, far away from the combat zone, I was having a pleasant chat.

'You're a wonderful doctor,' said Joe, 'wonderful, wonderful, I don't know what I'd do without you.'

'Well, yes, of course,' I agreed, looking down to the frenzy of activity at the bottom of the bed, where there was an ever-growing pile of discarded bandages and dressings, under which the nurse, by now, had disappeared; I sensed some disapproval emanating from beneath it.

'That's what we're here for,' I said, cranking it up the saintliness a bit further just for the hell of it. 'To cure sometimes, but comfort always.'

'Wonderful people, doctors,' echoed Joe, steam beginning to rise from the pile.

I thought, being a wonderful doctor and all, that I should make at least a token effort to help and demonstrate that

I didn't consider simple manual labour to be beneath me. I picked up Joe's slippers and stooped to put one on. Slippers can be awkward things to the untrained: the Velcro clasp wouldn't come loose properly, and I couldn't get the heel on. Joe began to squirm, unwilling to criticise Dr Wonderful.

The nurse regarded my clumsy efforts with a gleam of satisfaction in her eye.

'That's the wrong foot,' she said.

Footnote: Dedicated to my nursing colleagues, particularly Rose Carragher and Kathleen McNally

A time for reflection

GP 3 October 2014

I love the autumn; it appeals to my sense of guilt, all those long summer evenings when I should have been doing something, but somehow never got round to doing it (I blame my catholic upbringing, we specialise in guilt, but then I blame it for everything, especially my sexual perversity).

Instead I can look forward to mid-winter's homely comforts; sitting in a comfortable armchair with a cup of hot cocoa while the wind howls outside and raindrops spatter on the window-pane, reading the great Russian novelists or surfing on-line porn.

House-calls are a joy at this time of year; today I drove along leaf-strewn country lanes as the woods turned to shimmering gold, spider webs festooning the hawthorns, besparkled with morning dew.

On impulse, I stopped and got out, ignoring the old woman in a black pointy hat who walked past, giving me the evil eye; witches or not, they still don't like being refused an antibiotic for their 'awful' cough.

I leaned on a roadside fence, a moment of reflection, a brief time for tranquillity, after a morning surgery which had been like a series of collisions. Somewhere a lonely curlew howled, or possibly it was a badger – I'm a little hazy on zoology. All was quiet, a peaceful, almost Arcadian scene (although most Arcadian scenes include nymphs and satyrs having a great time, if you know what I mean) and if W.B. Yeats had popped up from behind a bush gently wittering on about fairies I wouldn't have been a bit surprised; 'I am lone Lady Quietness, my sweet/And on this loomband I weave thy destiny.'

And then I thought, I should really be getting on with that emergency call, hope the CPR is going OK.

An encounter with Reynard

BMJ 13 September 1997

Home visits remain a pleasant and sociable part of rural general practice. There is a daily closeness to nature, which I think our colleagues in the cities and towns miss out on; the sense of order, of renewal and change, of rhythm, that gift which, as C S Lewis observed, allows us to celebrate both the joys of novelty and familiarity at the same time.

In the teeth of winter the snowdrops, then the crocuses; by March the daffodils; April ushers in the transient fragility of the cherry and magnolia blossoms; early May is the best time, meadows lush and fresh and moist with bluebells and morning dew. After that it gets a bit hectic,

June busting out all over, wild parties, weeds in wheels shooting long and low and lush.

But as usual in my life experience, there is a Dark Side to this bucolic existence, and a closeness to nature presumes its own responsibilities.

Last night, as I was driving home from a house call, a Hunter's Moon was gleaming down and the mist was luminous in the headlights. A cat ran in front of the car; as to me the only good cat is a squashed cat I didn't shirk my duty. I put the foot down and awaited the satisfying squelch of a confirmed kill, and only realised too late that it was in fact a young fox. It was under the wheels in a second. And I love foxes; I love their wildness, their feistiness, their sparkiness, the way their eyes shine in the starlight.

I stopped and got out to see something very distressing; the fox was squirming madly in the middle of the road, its eyes bloody with pain and fear and ruin, its hind legs dragging uselessly. I'd obviously given it a serious spinal injury. It was late at night and the little creature and I were alone; I knew what I had to do.

I lifted it off the road, although it was trying to bite me, took the wheel jack from my boot, and crushed its skull with one swipe. It was brutal stuff, and I had to keep my eyes open all the while, as it was a moving target and I could not bear to miss and have to try again; 'One shot,' just as Robert De Niro said in 'The Deer Hunter.'

Like most doctors I've often had to administer drugs in that twilight zone of relieving symptoms while possibly or probably hastening death, but I don't recall any of them disturbing me as much as having to kill that little fox so bloodily with my bare hands. Those actions were aseptic, surgical; the violence is invisible, unacknowledged, cloaked.

I wonder how much being removed in this way from the actual act diminishes the import of what it is we are actually doing. If euthanasia involved smashing somebody's skull, would anyone admit to 50 successful swings?

Footnote; As you will see below, this column generated a significant degree of controversy; abusive letters by the sack load from as far away as Tokyo, an article in the *Independent*, even a visit from the cops. But since I was allowed right of reply I was paid double that month – nice.

Dear Editor—Liam Farrell writes graphically about his brutal killing of a fox which he had crippled by deliberately driving over it. He seems to feel regret but no remorse for this act. Indeed, he invites our admiration: for his willingness to discharge the responsibilities he carries by virtue of his closeness to nature (pause for purple prose) and for his understanding of the wider issues raised by his behaviour (pause for second rate philosophising about euthanasia).

We wondered if we had missed the point. Was hitting the animal really accidental? If so, why the deceit? Black humour? An obscure attempt at irony? We decided not. The article isn't remotely funny, and Farrell is too self-regarding to be ironical. If the story is true we must conclude that its author is wilfully cruel to animals and insensitive to the feelings of people who might be affected by his actions. These are unappealing characteristics, and distressing to find in a doctor.

The Views and Reviews section is meant to be provocative, but we found this article deeply offensive. It is not right that space should be given to people to parade their vices in this self-indulgent and confrontational manner. Our view is that it would do the *BMJ* no harm to seek a replacement contributor forthwith.

BMJ apologises to cats everywhere

BMJ 11 October 1997

We have received over 50 letters complaining about Liam Farrell's piece and one letter supporting his dislike of cats. This is almost as many letters as we received when we got Mozart's birthday wrong and advocated an elaborate treatment for weaver fish stings when they can actually be treated with any warm fluid, including urine. The *BMJ* is not anticat (we have even debated getting an office cat), and we apologise to cats everywhere and to readers who were distressed by Liam's piece. He is a writer who might be called a 'magical realist,' and we hoped that readers would not take his writing literally. When the nursery rhyme describes cows jumping over the moon and dishes running away with spoons, neither cows nor dishes are intended to follow the advice. Similarly we implore readers not to squash cats.—Editor

Give a dog a bad name

BMJ 11 October 1997

Writing a column for the *BMJ* is both a great privilege and an onerous duty. Over 100 000 doctors from all across the world constitute an unparalleled arena in which to project my prejudices and lament my uncertainties. But writing for a journal which is already at the cutting edge of medical progress is a daunting challenge. How do I make my column stand out amid all this medical excellence? How do I shout loud enough that my voice be heard, because shouting too loud can be a perilous jade.

I write by stream of consciousness; the quirk, the caprice, the knights-move thought, the harsh imagery, something to grab the reader and make them read on and assimilate the message. And sometimes this can be too successful; the medium becomes the message, and the outré quote, the perverse jest commands all the attention and becomes a literary cuckoo; the real theme of the article gets shoved out of the nest, flops to the ground below and gets eaten by the local cat (perhaps I'm drawing this analogy too far). So from a writer's point of view the offending article was a failure; my purpose, to illustrate the brutal gravity of the act of mercy killing, became obscured and submerged in a dispute about cats.

I'm also a wee bit sorry for causing offence, which was not my intent; I recognise that some sincere and gentle-hearted people do genuinely possess excessively tender feelings towards cats.

But I'm not that sorry; where's your sense of humour? Have you never heard of poetic licence? The Theatre of the Absurd? When Jerry sticks Tom's head in a microwave oven do you complain? The vets and lay people who harangued me may have no understanding of the role of black humour in medical survival, but I would have expected more perspicacity from my colleagues; I received so much vituperative correspondence that there was hardly enough room in my surgery to swing a tabby.

So mea culpa, I confess that I've never actually driven deliberately over a live cat; for one thing they're too darned nippy (unless the cat has ME) and drink has slowed down my reflexes, and for another they're too busy out there in the wild killing 80 million native birds every year and disrupting the balance of nature. When did you last walk in the meadows and listen to the call of the corncrake?

This world is a strange, bewildering, and dangerous place. I can take an extreme liberal stance on abortion, euthanasia, and legalising drugs, brace myself for rural Ireland's reactionary backlash, and receive only thoughtful responses; I can write bitterly critical articles about the Provisional IRA, and when I stand back to dodge the bullets I instead receive polite reproof. Yet sling in a little offhand joke about driving over a cat and I find I've really stepped in a poodle; I trust that the Cat's Protection League does not have a paramilitary wing.

But I am in honourable company; Salman Rushdie and his Fatwa, me and my Catwa.

Not really a lie...

GP 2 September 2015

Soccer has become a sporting juggernaut, dwarfing all its competitors into insignificance. The wall-to-wall media coverage, the 24-hour hype, the colossal wages; Messi and Ronaldo earn enough each year to keep the average small dialysis unit going for, like, two minutes.

But a word of warning; sporting fashions come and go. I remember in the seventies show-jumping was big, the plummy tones of Raymond Brookes-Ward droning on about Mr Softee and Pennword Forge Mill and Annelly Drummond-Haye. Harvey Smith was infamous enough to have a rude gesture named after him.

We completed our final exams to a soundtrack of Syd Waddell eulogising the unforgettable Jocky Wilson as he sprinted to the World Darts championship. And where are they now? Darts and showjumping, relegated to Eurosport along with the synchronised swimming.

Snooker is also yesterday's sport, but in the eighties, as a young doc, I was once called to a middle-aged man with chest pain. Gasping in an armchair, his pain was central, crushing and radiating to his left arm; if it had been any more classical, Beethoven would have composed a symphony about it.

'You're having a heart attack,' I said. 'We need to get you to hospital as soon as possible.'

'I can't,' he whispered, gazing at something over my shoulder. Only then did I notice that snooker was on TV, Julio the Whirlwind against The Cockney Geezer.

Perhaps it was more than just the Geezer snookering the Whirlwind behind the pink; perhaps timor mortis exultat me, the immediacy of possible death had revealed starkly the transience of life, and the importance of living in the now, of relishing every moment. As Achilles said, 'Everything is more beautiful because we are doomed'.

'I can't,' he repeated. 'I have to watch the end of this match.'

It was a tricky situation; to let him die, or renege on my ethical obligations to truth and integrity.

But dissimulation is a skill every family doctor must learn (I never condone lying to patients, except when I do it, naturally).

'Don't worry,' I said. 'They'll have Sky TV in the coronary care unit.'

The good doctor

BMJ 28 September 2002

How do you define the good doctor? How do you solve a problem like Maria? Being kind and compassionate is all very well but we need more, the rage to achieve, the pride not to accept defeat; like Milton's Satan, our vices are indistinguishable from our virtues. The qualities demanded are multiple, and they fluctuate with time and circumstances.

Jennie had an unusual form of high spirited and happy dementia, and just as I arrived at the farm she was bolting out through the door, over the wall and across the fields. Her family came tumbling out after, but seeing I had arrived, they stopped and looked at me expectantly, like the Council of Elrond looking at Frodo and thinking, 'Here comes a real sucker, problem solved.'

But being A Good Doctor, I accepted the metaphorical baton and set off in pursuit, leaping the wall and tipping over the other side, though luckily my fall was cushioned by some broken bottles. I could see Jennie in the distance, a glimmering girl fading in the brightening air among long dappled grass, dodging behind the dread vista of a fine herd of Jersey cows.

The cows represented a serious escalation. If you are ever hunted by the law, and have to escape across the fields, choose a field with cows. City folk mightn't appreciate this, but cows are intelligent creatures and get bored standing around in the field all day. During the Troubles, when the British Army were on patrol, taking cover at the side of a field, the cows would wander over to have a look. So anytime you saw a line of cows staring into a ditch, you knew where the soldiers were hiding.

An exciting chase is an even more welcome diversion, so the herd galloped over for a better look. The avoidance of stampeding cows is not something we are taught in medical school, and I swiped at them uselessly with my black bag.

Distracted, I then trod in a cow pat so large and liquid that a small boy could swim in it. The quarry may not mind running through cow dung, but the sartorial demands of our profession leave us ill equipped for this task. And once dung gets on your clothes, the smell will endure forever; trust me on this point.

I caught Jennie at the far end of the field.

'Ah, doctor,' she said playfully, as I grabbed her desperately by the ear, 'I thought you'd never catch me.'

A good doctor is a doctor who can run fast and is not over-fastidious regarding personal hygiene. QED.

Footnote: The BMJ ran a theme issue on 'what makes a good doctor,' and I was requested to make my usual thoughtful contribution.

Chapter 13

Hospital life

Gracie and I, in paediatric outpatients, alone; except for two clown doctors. Disturbing enough, but the true horror was about to dawn. A nurse appeared to sweep Gracie off for an x-ray.

Now it was just me and the clowns, who were really professional; no chance of them nipping out for a smoke-break or taking off their false noses. They steadfastly remained in character, taking pratfalls, making funny faces, while I began to hyperventilate.

So that's what hospital means to me; clowns ... and nightmares

A rapid promotion

GP 1 October 2008

When I was a surgical intern in Dublin, my six months of torture and ritualised humiliation included a short rotation as a gynaecology intern. As the consultant was never around - that's private medicine for you - and the reg was flaky, I became the de facto gynae expert in the hospital, Suddenly, I was doing consults all around the hospital; suddenly, I was The Man Who Knew. No-one else was comfortable with incontinence, prolapses, inserting ring pessaries, etc, so my own incompetence in these areas was easy to cover up; in the country of the blind (and stupid) the one-eyed gynae intern is king.

But, sometimes, I had to call outside help. One of our pre-op patients developed toothache, a complex condition obviously beyond my expertise.

'Call the dental team,' I was advised by a helpful nurse.

'We have a dental team? Since when? Do a lot of people know that?' I was shocked that such a thing existed but, in the noble tradition of junior doctors since time immemorial, eager to seize the opportunity of fobbing the problem off on some other poor sap. It's recognised as sound medical practice.

I called the switchboard.

'Can you contact the dental team for me?' I asked.

'No problem,' they said reassuringly, like they'd done it hundreds of times before.

A few seconds later my bleep went off.

'You're wanted in gynae,' was the message.

'I'm already here,' I replied, looking round at the speculae on the shelf just to make sure.

'Good, because the gynae intern wants you to see somebody.'

'There must be some mistake,' I said, 'I am the gynae intern, why would I be looking for myself?'

There was a brief silence, then rustling papers, suggesting a list was being checked.

'Congratulations,' they said - could I hear giggling? 'You're the dental intern as well.'

'Quite a promotion,' I said, 'I'll just ask myself for my own opinion then, shall I?'

The giggles turned to cackles; 'Just don't bite off more than you can chew, Dental Boy.'

Making technology work (for me)

GP 23 May 2012

When I was a junior doctor in a rural hospital, the local community had been fundraising for years for an ultrasound scanner, which back in the early eighties was the very latest thing. Eventually, after innumerable guest teas and raffles and sponsored walks and beard-shaves and circumcisions, a new machine was purchased for £10,000, a lot of money in those days. An ultrasound scan was at that time every patient's dream, and to point out that it would be bugger-all use would have been an unpopular stance.

People came from miles to see it, and being the size of a small house, it was an impressive sight. All bells and whistles, it seemed to be at the cutting edge of science; 'like walking on the moon', a man described it, a man whose surname, coincidentally, was Mooney.

Trouble was, no one knew how to use it; the radiologist was about a thousand years old, show him anything but a chest X-ray and he'd get confused and forget his own name, and there was no money to employ a new one. So the scanner was stuck in the high-tech room, the purpose of which was to look like a high-tech room, as if high-tech stuff was being done there; in fact nothing ever got done, we just kept stuff.

But I learned from this experience that Knowledge is Power, and a few years later I was senior house officer (well, acting registrar, really) in a special care baby ward when a new-fangled state-of-the-art monitoring device was delivered.

As the only doc there at the time, the rep showed me how to use it, and I hoarded this information jealously, becoming the de facto expert. My street-cred went up like a rocket, and from being the lowest of the low in the pecking order, I was launched into the stratosphere, and bestrode the hospital like a pudgy, prematurely balding colossus.

Not a day would pass without me getting an urgent call because the machine was honking in distress. Usually it was something ridiculously simple, but for the sake of my reputation, I always put on a proper theatrical show for my audience; thoughtful expression, furrowed brow, twiddling knobs and pressing buttons like I was splitting the atom.

As a bonus I used to throw in a bit of implied criticism of my colleagues. Nothing too overt, just a subtle tut-tut, a raising of a laconic eyebrow, or occasionally, 'You mean they haven't calibrated it?' Undermining other junior doctors was an essential ingredient of career progression in those days; what fun we had. If the audience was sufficiently gullible, which was pretty often, I'd throw in a few cryptic remarks about oxygen saturation or CO_2 levels.

Oddly, the more senior the audience, the easier the sell. The consultants were dear old chaps; they meant well, bless their hearts, but they were utterly baffled by the advance of science.

'When you see the red light blinking,' I'd explain patiently (because I was always taught to humour old folks), 'that means the machine is on.'

'It's wonderful,' old Bonzo would say, scratching his woolly head in bewilderment.

And it was also a brilliant excuse for skiving off work. If there was an influx of admissions, while everyone else was busy as bees, I'd be found on the machine, doing the knob thing and inspecting print-outs with magisterial diligence.

On the last day, I had to choose my successor; I spotted him at once, chewing gum morosely at the back of the orientation class. There's a likely lad, I thought, he could do with a leg-up.

'Use this gift wisely, grasshopper,' I told him.

I'll have mine rare

GP 27 Sept 2013

As the Fat Man said in *The House of God*, when a medical student hears hoof-beats outside a window, he thinks it's a zebra. Which might be true, of course, in certain circumstances, like if you were in practice in the Serengeti (although curiously, I was once in the Serengeti, heard hoof-beats outside my window, peered out through the early morning mist and saw only an old cow; I've always been lucky that way).

Because common things are common, and uncommon presentations of common diseases are more common that common presentations of uncommon diseases. But sometimes….

As an intern I saw a young lad in casualty. He had fainted at a disco (yes, it was that long ago, *Saturday Night Fever* was quite fashionable, old age is creeping up on me, not sure why but I'm fairly sure it's up to no good), had a few unusual skin lesions and a labile blood pressure. Nowadays I wouldn't recognise a phaeochromocytoma if one walked up and assaulted me with a blunt speculum (I've matured since, been flogged into apathy by too many URTIs and sick certs; rare and interesting diseases only present to other doctors), but I was young then,

314

fresh and sharp and so hip I could hardly see over my pelvis.

I wrote in the chart '?possible neurofibromatosis? possible phaeo?' and admitted him to the ward. I was too green to realise the importance of hoarding unusual cases to myself, for my own advancement, and sure enough, the rumour spread around the hospital as fast as an epidemic of flaming gonorrhea.

When I went to check up on my patient later, I found him buried beneath a red tide of medical students, SHOs and research registrars, all keen for a piece of the glory, all ordering 24 hr urines to beat the band, all dreaming of a case report for the peer-reviewed journals (not the important ones, of course, but any port in a storm) and another notch on their CVs.

'Help doc,' he said desperately, 'They're suffocating me.'

I whipped away the medical students, but the others were far above me in the hierarchy, and I could offer little succour.

'Sorry pal,' I said, 'It's a common complication of uncommon diseases.'

Cometh the hour, cometh the doc....

GP 15 January 2010

When I was a lad, medicine was still adhering slavishly to the traditional doctrine that the sickest and most vulnerable patients should be looked after by the most inexperienced and incompetent doctors; casualty consultants were unheard of and the other consultants would have laughed at them anyway. Casualty then was sleeves rolled up, blood and muck to the knees, finger in the dyke stuff, and Saturday nights were like a war zone.

One night I was the only doctor on duty when the fight started, usually my signal to instantly flee (hey, someone had to tell the outside world). Go Tell the Spartans, I thought nobly, but unfortunately, I had delayed too long, and the fight had already mushroomed and spilled throughout the department. All egress was blocked, what was a guy to do?

But learning to improvise is all part of a doctor's training.

I grabbed a baby from a cot and, holding it up like a talisman, began to thread my way through the mayhem, pausing only to wipe some blood from a passing meatcleaver and smear it on my face. The long-term risk of hepatitis B was a poor second to the short-term risk of brutal dismemberment.

'Watch out for the baby!' I shouted; the baby, obviously having read the script, and being a good baby, began to cry piteously.

Bursting through the doors into the main hospital, I realised a crowd had gathered, and that I cut a rather dashing figure. I also knew that a little bit of theatre was called for.

'Someone take the baby,' I said, with an air of weary heroism, 'I gotta go back in'.

Hands grabbed at me, just as I had planned.

'You can't go back in, it's madness, you're bleeding,' chanted the crowd.

'You don't understand,' I protested, the very picture of agonised and conflicted virtue, 'there may be more babies in there.'

I struggled to escape their clutches; but didn't struggle too hard, of course.

Medical conceits; the Grand Round

GP 3 September 2008

I received some spam a few weeks ago, inviting me to purchase some little blue pills with apparently wondrous qualities and another to subscribe to a 'grand' round; before deletion, I circulated them to all the people I don't like. But it did bring back some happy memorics.

When I was a student in Dublin, our professor decided to institute a 'grand' round. Even in those more innocent days (and Ireland was very innocent then), this was largely recognised for the conceit it was, a way of reminding all the other consultants that though they earned far more money than him and had bigger shinier cars (this is important to consultants, especially the *emeritus* ones), due to their private practice, they still yearned for academic respectability and he was still the biggest dog in the yard.

On the first day of the 'grand' round, the requisite crowd turned up, a mixture of sulky consultants, slobbering registrars eager for advancement, baffled SHOs, exhausted interns, and hungover medical students, all waiting in fascination for the disasters that we knew were certain to ensue.

The big problem was that our professor was not very popular with patients, so when the hordes swept in to the first ward only one little old lady (LOL) was in bed. The senior registrar presented the not-very-interesting case, after which the whole troupe shuffled outside to discuss it in the corridor.

I was at the back of the crowd, so I couldn't hear very much, not that I cared, the bits that I could pick up concerned mostly her bowel movements and how normal they were, when I noticed the nurse wheeling the above

LOL out of the first ward. Sure enough, when we entered the second ward, there she was again, gloriously alone.

Then, to our eternal delight, one of the registrars who had arrived late and missed the first ward, started presenting the case again. Most of the crowd, his competitors, were more than happy for him to keep digging, while other more decent souls did try to gain his attention, making furtive cutting throat gestures, but this was his moment in the sun, his big day, nothing was going to stop him, and he continued to the bitter end.

When he at last finished there was a long silence, punctuated only by the sniggers of the medical students.

'Any questions?' asked the prof, looking as deflated as the consultants were smug.

'Can I go home?' said the LOL.

My very own Guardian Angel

GP 11 July 2017

My sister was admitted to Moorfields Eye Hospital in London a few weeks ago, receiving brachytherapy for a retinal melanoma. The procedure went very well, and I can't speak highly enough of Moorfields and the team on the observation ward; they were endlessly kind and thoroughly professional, the NHS at its best.

While the radioactive plate was in situ, my sister was radioactive, so, being a doctor and therefore immune to radiation, I was delegated by the family to keep an eye on her, so to speak.

In sunny weather I wear a pair of wrap-around shades that fit conveniently over my normal specs. On the first day, while going into the hospital, I stumbled slightly. The man behind caught my arm and asked if I was OK.

I reassured him I was fine, then he asked me where I was going.

'Fourth floor,' I said.

'I'll take you there,' he said, which was very decent of him; the first time in a new hospital it can be hard to find your way around, and like Blanche Dubois, I have always been dependent on the kindness of strangers. But as we were walking along, he took me gently by the arm, and it slowly dawned on me, because (1) the stumble, (2) the shades and (3) the context, he thought I was visually impaired.

By this time he had escorted me to the lift and I felt it would be impolite and inconsiderate to suddenly whip off the shades say, 'no look, I can see great'; I was so steeped in gore that to go back were as bloody as to go o'er.

'Thanks, I'll be fine now,' I said, but my Guardian Angel was not to be deterred and insisted on waiting with me to make sure I got into the lift without a calamity. There followed an interminably long wait, by which time a queue had gathered, some obviously with a genuine visual impairment.

Eventually the lift arrived.

'Step back, please,' my GA announced. 'Let this gentleman on first.'

I walked into the lift, fumbling theatrically at the buttons, as if I was identifying the number 4 by touch.

'So brave,' murmured someone behind me.

My GA waited till the doors were closing and waved me a last goodbye.

And, damn it, before I could stop myself, I waved back.

Believe it or not

BMJ 1 March 2007

Belief is an emotional state that is not susceptible to rational persuasion, said Spinoza. And, boy, could I sing a few bars of that—although my seminal experience was not at some frenzied religious festival with people slashing themselves theatrically or falling down speaking in tongues but in the cold light of the surgical ward.

When I was a surgical intern a young man was admitted with a left upper quadrant mass. Ireland was a poor country then; advanced imaging was not available, so the diagnosis largely depended on clinical examination and was a mystery until the senior registrar arrived.

'It's an enlarged spleen,' he proclaimed, 'I can feel a notch.'

His certainty was such that none could gainsay him. We all had another go; sure enough, there it was clear as a day: a notch. How could we have missed it?

The news spread like wildfire around the hospital and further afield. Medical students just love their clinical signs, and they came in their thousands to palpate this wonderful notch. The senior registrar, by now rather proprietorial, would, with the touch of a showman, gently guide their hands over the patient's abdomen. They would palpate timidly, seem confused and uncertain—but then, as they looked at the senior registrar's expectant face, their eyes would light up. 'Yes, there it is, I can feel it, it's a notch, most definitely a notch, a wonderful, wonderful notch, the most wonderful notch that I have ever felt.'

It was a bandwagon: the enthusiasm was infectious and overwhelming. As with the emperor's new clothes, no one wanted to be an outsider; everyone wanted to belong, to be part of the gang. Everyone either believed they really could feel that notch or pretended they could, in case they looked stupid.

Our senior registrar's stock rose mightily. The message was clear, he opined grandly to his adoring acolytes, like a fat and obnoxious Buddha: blood tests and x-rays are all very well, but at the end of the day you couldn't beat good old-fashioned clinical acumen.

Dawn came up like thunder on the fatal conclave, the day of the laparotomy, the gallery packed with supporters. We opened up the patient and found ... a big kidney and, to add insult to injury, a small and rather apologetic spleen. The senior registrar paled, the crowd sagged, detumescent with disappointment, and at the back someone started singing;

'The king is in the altogether, the altogether ...'

Fond memories of the Journal Club

GP 3 April 2015

If I miss anything about the ritual humiliations of being a junior doctor (apart from the rampant promiscuity, which became quite onerous after a while, but some medical conventions simply must be observed), it's the Journal Club.

Was anything ever so restful? It was just the thing for an exhausted junior; grab a coffee, sit at the back and be lulled to sleep by the stumbling presentation of the unfortunate (and usually unwilling) presenter.

So Plod's appearance at the Journal Club drew a big crowd, all in search of a quick nap.

Plod originally acquired his nickname because of his initials, but in what was an incredible cosmic accident, or because he felt compelled to grow into the role, 'Plod' summed him up very neatly.

He was slow, yet dull, and spoke in a soporific monotone. But as Soren Kierkegaard observed, 'What labels me, negates me,' and Plod was ready to confound our expectations.

He stood up at the front and, ignoring the gentle sounds of snoring (the junior residence wasn't exactly the Algonquin Round Table) began to draw an exquisitely detailed diagram of the inner ear. Michelangelo would have been less perfectionist painting the Sistine Chapel.

Plod had been given 30 minutes, but after 20, we were only halfway through the cochlea and the postgrad tutor was becoming agitated.

The crowd roused from its slumber; could he finish the 30 minutes without actually speaking a word? And as the time-limit ticked past, Plod ended with a rebellious smile.

'Voila,' he said, 'the inner ear.'

Plod's demonstration was a metaphor for a deeper truth - the danger of labels. A diagnosis minimises patients; even the term 'patient' does many-faceted individuals an injustice.

The postgrad tutor was most disgruntled, but, as is mandatory, he was just a jumped-up, overly ambitious registrar, whom we all despised and made fun of .

Behind his back, of course; some medical conventions simply must be observed.

Good advice?

BMJ 6 July 2002

As with a tip for the horses, the responsibility for advice lies not with the donor but with the recipient; words are cheap, and ultimately it's your choice whether to act on them or not.

On my first night as casualty officer a young man was brought in unconscious. In those days I was quite thorough (I've matured since), so—among other things (such as pressing knuckles on his sternum to check he wasn't faking)—I ordered a drug screen.

I then received a call from the lab technician who explained politely that it was not lab policy to perform drug screens on unconscious patients without certain other indications. They had a protocol, she said. I can't remember what these indications were, but in those days, protocols were new-fangled and sounded quite impressive.

In those days, also, I was easily persuadable (I've matured since), which is usually a virtue and especially so in Northern Ireland, so I accepted this explanation. But when I described what had happened over coffee to the medical registrar, who'd been working there for donkey's years, he bristled with rage.

'I'm sick of those bastards,' he said, 'What do lab techs know about patient care? That guy is your patient, you are the doctor, you are on the front line, you make the decisions; you are responsible, if something goes wrong, it won't be the lab tech who gets the blame. The buck stops with you, and if you think you need a drug screen, damn well order it;' it was pretty rousing stuff.

Once again easily persuaded (sometimes this is not such a virtue), I rang back the lab tech and damn well ordered the drug screen done stat, with no arguments and no messing, right? I was the doctor, he was my patient etc. A few minutes later, the casualty sister came in and, portentously discreet, whispered deafeningly and rather moistly in my ear that the professor of chemical pathology wanted to speak to me at once.

'F***,' said the reg, making the traditional medical handwashing gesture, 'You're in big trouble now.'

Footnote; A true story.

The good slut

BMJ 12 August 2004

Call me Ishmael; I wander in the desert, eating locusts, eluding hostile nomads, and sucking on spit. I am a general practitioner, I prowl in the night, perilous and alone. I meet the old and the lost, the desperate and the lonely.

I know how you feel, the despair, the hopelessness. A home visit, the house is cold and damp, a pervading smell of stale urine and mildew. No food in the fridge, an old kettle and stale bread and teabags in the kitchen.

No hot water. Night isn't just falling, more like sharpening its claws. The elderly woman is frail, isolated, frightened, no family or friends.

There's nothing overtly medical wrong with her, but social services are far, far away; it's just you and her, and you think to yourself, 'Fuck it, she can't stay here, I have to do something.' And in my darkest and most dreadful hours I may call for help, for I know there is one friend who will always answer my call.

'Send her on in,' said the medical senior house officer, in a tone weary with resignation and suffering; I wanted to give him a big hug.

The acute medical ward is the slut of medicine; it'll take on anyone, anytime, and it is the place of last resort. This is a good thing, and a most honourable calling. What your patient needs right now is a hot bath, a decent meal, a comfortable bed and some human kindness. A gentle touch, the brush of a human hand, the silent, reflex-level affirmation that someone is near, that someone cares; a refuge, a sanctuary against the cold and the darkness.

But the NHS has no overt facility for this kind of acute care, hospitals like to think of themselves as high-tech centres of excellence, dealing with fancy stuff, diabetic keto-acidoses, thyrotoxic crises, transplants, big trauma.

Social reasons aren't supposed to be grounds for admission, so part of the ritual is that the family doctor then has to construct a flimsy Trojan horse of plausible medical grounds to access this care. Our moral compromise is slow but implacable, and such invention and dissimulation become easy with practice; so many illnesses accompany neglect that it is only a matter of choosing the handiest one.

So our admission letters are not downright lies; they are only half-truths, harmless little fibs in pursuit of the greater good.

Medical intervention, though a nice optional extra, is usually way down on the patient's list of needs, but the patient will still have to endure the charade of being quizzed, poked, and prodded as the unfortunate junior doctor has to play the game out to the bitter end.

And then, eventually, your patient will receive the care she needs.

Chapter 14

Death

In Ireland we have an ambivalent approach to death. Before it happens, we are defensive and guarded, and denial is our most popular coping mechanism. But after death (especially if it's somebody else's) our attitude changes radically, and we have what is known as a wake, a triumphant ceremony celebrating life in the face of death, an acceptance that death is a fitting end to what was a good story and a tale well worth the telling.

The death of a child or a young adult is never fair, never right, but for older people a wake can be a kind of posthumous This Is Your Life, and merriment and devilment of all kinds can ensue as we trade stories through the night about the deceased and their exploits.

Life was simple - you were born, you lived, you died. The swallows depart, the hawthorn bushes blush red-hued with crimson berries, Tiger Woods has a new ladyfriend, the leaves turn brown and golden, an abundance of metaphors for the transience of our lives. Life is precious, fleeting and ephemeral, and the difference between the living and the dead is only a matter of time.

But all is changed, utterly changed...

Death, where is thy sting?

BMJ 9 October 2003

I'm an old-fashioned general practitioner; Dr Finlay and I would have got on famously, gone out drinking together, maybe clubbing in Ibiza, etc. I still enjoy home visits, and value the precious insights gained from enjoying cups of tea and big slices of homemade apple pie in the kitchen with Granny Arbuckle, before drinking quarts of cider and sneaking off for a quick shag with her buxom niece Sally amid the fields of barley (OK, I made the last bit up; it seems such a logical progression).

But house calls aren't always fun, especially at a spooky time like Halloween.

The cottage was deep in the woods. As usual, on calls where the welcome is uncertain, I parked facing away from the house and on a down slope, and left the engine running, all to facilitate a quick getaway.

The countryside, so familiar during the day, seemed now veiled and threatening, and the menacing eyes of sheep loomed up on every side. You city folk think sheep are cuddly and innocent, but get between a pack of sheep and their prey, and you're in for a stomping.

The farmyard was guarded by a three-headed hound carrying a knife and fork, which struck me as curious yet apt. It snarled at me affectionately, but I placated it by stuffing my fingers up its nostrils until it suffocated; animals respond to kindness, don't you know.

The skeletal figure of Death sat in front of a waning fire. He pointed a bony finger at me.

'I have a task for you, doctor,' he said, in a tone that managed to be both sepulchral and whiny at the same time, 'I have an awful cough, and I thought maybe… an antibiotic?'

He hawked noisily and spat generously into the grate, only lightly spraying me on the way. There was a whoosh and sizzle, and the dying embers wrought their ghost upon the floor a month earlier than usual.

My clinical instincts are always alert, and I noticed from the specks on my silk cravat that his sputum was nonpurulent. I explained firmly that he had a viral illness, and he should rest and take plenty of fluids.

He sagged in disappointment, then perked up again.

'My back's giving me gyp,' he said, 'what about sending me for an x-ray?'

'Difficult,' I said, 'At this time of night there'll only be a skeleton staff on duty.'

An unusual approach to Advance Care Planning

GP   26 July 2017

Joe looked unusually pensive, which cheered me up a bit and added some sparkle to the morning.

'Your native hue of resolution / Is sicklied o'er with the pale cast of thought,' I observed.

'I was wondering,' said Joe, 'if I should get an advance care plan in place.'

I was a bit surprised by such a display of forethought, the first falling leaves of vulnerability; Joe has always been a man who demanded immediate gratification of all his desires, his only forward planning on the lines of how big a steak to eat tonight, or the most likely winner of the 3.30pm at Kilbeggan today.

'So what would you like in your advance care plan?' I said. 'I can give you a form with all the information.' I love giving out forms, it saves me having to explain every bloody thing myself, like I don't have, you know, a life.

'Most important thing,' he said. 'I want a big flat screen TV, with Sky Sports, the Racing Channel and Netflix.'

'We may have a misunderstanding here,' I said. 'An advance care plan is a legal document in which you specify what actions should be taken for your health if you are no longer able to make decisions for yourself. We should all have one signed and filed, to avoid having some big sweaty guy pounding gaily and unnecessarily on our chest. But what it will not specify is having a big TV in your room.'

Joe was undeterred by such minor details.

'When I'm dying,' he insisted, 'I want a big TV; pull the plug on me before you pull it on the TV.'

He gripped my hand urgently and looked me straight in the eyes.

'Can I trust you to do that for me, doc?' he said. 'Can I trust you not to pull the plug?'

Antibiotics, sick notes and the afterlife

GP 8 March 2016

I don't usually talk to The Dead, though I do have a soft spot for them; they're not covered by our contract, so we are not at their immediate beck and call, like we are for everyone else.

But Joe was an exception; just as in our consultations while he was alive, I knew he'd slobber and threaten and bluster and cry and whinge and whine until he eventually got his own way.

He was wearing the traditional ghostly white shift, though, being Joe, the white shift already looked a bit stretched and grubby. Tomato sauce stains streaked down the front, counterpointed by the fragrance of fried onions. Joe was obviously getting the kind of heaven he had always desired.

'I told you...' he started, then stopped.

'I TOLD YOU...' he continued, changing his timbre in an effort to appear more ghostly, obviously something they get taught on day one in Ghost School (in the same way that Surgical School encourages clipped tones, a big shiny car, and a smirk).

'Before you go on,' I interrupted, 'I know what you're going to say; 'I told you I was sick'. You needn't bother, Spike Milligan has already done it.'

'YEAH, YEAH, ALRIGHT,' he said, with a petulance not usually associated with the sepulchral tones of The Dead. 'BUT YOU SHOULD HAVE GIVEN ME AN ANTIBIOTIC; AND SENT ME FOR AN X-RAY.'

'So what can I do for you?' I said, the antibiotic prescription already half-written (it usually saves time).

'THERE'S NO DOCTORS HERE,' said Joe.

I speculated that (a) doctors don't get into heaven because the gods don't like us, or more likely (b) a doctor's heaven doesn't include patients like Joe.

'GOD INSISTS WE TURN UP REGULARLY FOR ADORATION AND WORSHIP AND STUFF, USU-ALLY WHEN THE HORSE RACING IS ON,' said Joe.

'Inconvenient,' I admitted.

'YEAH, IT CAN BE A REAL PAIN SOMETIMES - AND SHE DOESN'T LOOK A BIT LIKE MORGAN FREEMAN,' he said. 'SO, I WAS WONDERING, MAYBE A SICK NOTE?'

As on earth, so shall it be in heaven, I thought.

The silver lining

BMJ 6 October 2009

Each September, at Croke Park, when the ball is thrown in at the All-Ireland Gaelic Football final, every true Irishman's heart beats a little faster. It is our spiritual home, but for many years it had been a bitter vale of tears for County Armagh.

Until 2002. That year our team had a vigour, a sense of purpose—maybe this year would be different, maybe this year we would take the Sam Maguire Cup home for the very first time.

Orange and white flags and bunting festooned every house and lamp post; orange and white sheep grazed every field and meadow; a plaster orange and white cow patrolled the boreens. The frenzy grew as the big game drew near, and the ferocity of the scramble for tickets allowed no moral compass.

'I'm worried about Joe,' said Joe's brother.

'Indeed,' I said, sympathetic yet wary.

'It's terrible, terrible,' he said, shaking his head sadly, the very picture of fraternal grief; and then, suddenly shifty, 'He won't be fit to make the final then. He'll hardly need his ticket, will he?'

Like buzzards on a gut wagon, any sign of frailty was seized on, and even distant relatives became very attentive. Every time I visited Joe I'd see people surreptitiously opening drawers and checking out mantelpieces.

And all the machinations were made glorious summer by those sun-bursting moments when Oisin McConville sliced through the Kerry defence for the crucial goal and Kieran McGeeney raised the cup high in the air. Cut him out in little stars, we cried, and he shall make the face of heaven so fine that all the world shall fall in love with night; let there be dancing in the streets, drinking in the saloons, and necking in the parlours.

The glow lasted all through a golden autumn and a long and lustrous winter. Children born that year had naturally curly hair and a sunny disposition and were immune to papillovirus infections.

Death was no barrier to the glow, which provided consolation even at those times of deepest sorrow.

A few weeks after the match, at Joe's wake, I gathered the family.

'Wasn't he lucky: he lived long enough to see Armagh win the title,' I told them. 'Yeah, he was a great football man,' someone chipped in.

'Never missed a match,' we agreed, and sorrow and loss ebbed gently away as we sat all night happily talking about football, while the embers faded and the moon waned in the sky, the hour when death is like a light and blood is like a rose.

Thanks for the ticket, Joe, I thought.

Footnote; Papillovirus infection causes warts.

Footnote 2; I'm from County Down, and we hate Armagh

Breaking good news

BMJ 31 October 2012

'How long does granny have, doctor?'

'Only a few days,' I said. I was young and beautiful and too green to know that the wise clinician always fudges the prognosis. Within minutes the message was winging its way across the globe.

A few nights later and there were relatives tucked in every corner, swinging on the rafters, hanging from the roof, dangling from the curtains. They had ridden in on the four winds, swum dangerous rivers, climbed huge mountains, endured biting insects and even Ryanair flights. They'd come from Boston, Singapore, Sydney, Vladivostok, all determined to be there at granny's deathbed.

So I was disconcerted to find granny looking much better, quite perky even. Breaking bad news is all part of the job, but breaking good news was a novel challenge.

'I have good news,' I said, trying gamely to give it a positive spin, 'Your granny's not dying after all. She's looking much better. Ain't that great?'

There was an ominous silence, which, inexperienced as I was, I felt compelled to fill.

'Underneath it all, she has a great engine, heart like a lion, strong as a horse, and all,' I continued, starting to babble, hoping that this testament to the clan's animal virility might soften the blow.

'We were told she was very ill,' accused Boston.

A rebellious muttering began. 'It's cost me a bloody fortune,' from the deserts of Sudan. 'My return flight is next weekend,' from the gardens of Japan. 'I've taken a week off work for this,' from Milan. 'I knew there was bugger all wrong with her,' from Yucatan. The crowd shifted threateningly forward, as crowds do when someone has a rope, a nearby tree has a convenient low branch.

'Don't lose hope,' I said, 'I've adopted the Liverpool care pathway.'

Footnote; the Liverpool care pathway was an attempt to rationalise the treatment of dying patients e.g by withdrawing unnecessary medications. At this time, it was coming under attack; accusations were made that it was simply a way of saving money.

Footnote 2; this column, based almost nearly on a true story, received mixed responses, such as...

Dear Editor

Re: Breaking good news

I initially thought that this would be an excellent piece - outlining the professional dilemma when prognosis turns out not to be as expected or predicted. Unfortunately, the last sentence of the piece ruins what could have been a thought-provoking reflective essay and transforms it into a dreadful piece of writing by an ill-informed individual and written in very bad taste.

Experienced and informed professionals specialising in end of life care, and the many more generalists who provide significant amounts of similar care, are currently struggling to reassure their patients and the public that end of life care can be appropriate and of a high quality, despite the recent scaremongering tactics about the LCP by second-rate journalists. Dr Farrell adds nothing to the debate and, in fact, potentially causes great harm through his writing by, barely obliquely, suggesting that the LCP can be used to end a patient's life.

I view this as contemptible, irresponsible and unprofessional behaviour, and do hope that Dr Farrell takes the time to learn more about the LCP or, if he has done so previously, realises that he needs re-training in its principles and use.

Dear Editor

Re: Breaking good news

Boy this guy can write! Loved it. Hilariously puncturing delusions of medical omniscience. I took reference to LCP as great satire on recent coverage. More from Dr Farrell please.

Saying goodbye with a favourite song

GP 18 September 2015

Doctors are like the great novelists, 'in' a situation, but not 'of' it. We can stand back, observe, and enjoy the entertainment.

The relatives were gathered round the death-bed like buzzards. Grandad had led a long, fulfilling and (very) fruitful life, and was going gently into the good night. Dylan Thomas would have been most disappointed, but the many fruits of his loins weren't going to let him go quietly; that's not the Irish Way, they'd flown in from all corners of the world for the occasion and were going to get their moneys-worth.

One-upmanship is rife at these gatherings. In one corner, arrangements were being made for the funeral, negotiations of Cold War delicacy; who would carry the coffin (and in what order), who would give the readings; the hierarchy of grief had to be observed.

As ever, the more geographically distant relatives were the most demanding, over-compensating for the fact they hadn't seen the old chap for years; the traditional divisive family argument, sure to be handed down the generations, was inevitable.

There was a near fatality when Singapore fell off the end of the bed (prime real estate in these circumstances), and

Argentina nipped in to take a quick selfie. But as attrition rates go at such volatile conclaves, one casualty wasn't bad.

'Let's all sing Grandad's favourite hymn,' said Toronto, and he started to croon something about St Patrick and the Good Shepherd sharing a joint. But he was on his own. 'Does nobody know the words?' he said, feigning distress, but actually quite smug.

'We'll Google it,' said Silicon Valley, and the group huddled around the laptop, the glow of the screen lending the room a ghostly light.

The lyrics were located and the singing started; but there was disagreement over the melody, so YouTube was searched. Multiple fingers poking clumsily at computer keys, and *Slippery when Wet* boomed out, closely flowed by *Sexual Healing*.

Eventually the right song was located; the crowd listened for a while, picking up the tune, then joined in enthusiastically.

'The teachers always said he was very bright,' said the proud mum of Silicon Valley.

'By the way,' I said. 'Grandad died a few minutes ago.'

The dance of death

BMJ 24 July 2012

'So,' I asked, 'how did it happen?'

'Well,' he said, 'I was at a wedding and I got up to dance—that's when I felt the pain in my chest.'

I was curious; for the third time in a matter of weeks a man in his 50s had had a myocardial infarct while at a wedding. The risk factors were obvious: overweight, unfit, suddenly hurled into intense physical activity, but could there be something more going on, something sinister?

'What song was the band playing at the time?' I asked. The experienced clinician knows that the devil is in the details.

'*Dancing Queen,*' he said. 'And what can you do? It was like an outside force taking over my body—my feet started tapping, my hips twitching, resistance is futile, I just had to join in.'

'Dull would he be of soul who could pass by,' I agreed.

On a hunch, I pulled the files, made a few calls, and, sure enough, on each occasion *Dancing Queen* had been playing. The potency of cheap music, I reflected. Noël Coward was right.

Then, with a chill of horror, I realised that there was another wedding on that very day.

I dashed out of the surgery and drove headlong to the reception, almost running down a lady with long blonde hair and a curiously appropriate spangly, sparkly jumpsuit.

'*Se vart du ska*, idiot,' she said.

'*Du kysser din mamma med den munnen?*' I inquired ('You kiss your mother with that mouth?')—I'd picked up a smattering of Swedish during my years as a Euro-trash porn star.

I burst in through the door just as the song was reaching a climax with that immortal, almost Shakespearean lyric, 'Feel the beat of the tambourine, OH *YEAH* . . .'

As the crowd punched the air in a pagan frenzy, a short fat man collapsed on the floor. I cradled his head in my arms, as he whispered his dying words: 'Diggin' . . . the dancing queen . . .'

'Damn you, Benny Andersson and Björn Ulvaeus, damn you,' I cried, shaking my fist at the heavens.

But in time with the beat, of course.

Footnote; my niece Ros, out of whose eyes the stars shine, married Ben a few years ago. Their wedding was a wonderful, unforgettable day, made doubly so by Uncle Rory inspiring this column.

A-wake?

BMJ 26 April 1997

A great old patient of mine was dying recently and I told his wife that he might not last till morning, promising that I would come back to put him down for the night. When I returned I had to park over a mile away up the boreen, such was the throng. Passing the kitchen, I felt a blast of wild fiddle music, whiskey fumes, and boisterous laughter that nearly knocked me flat. There was even a Fat Lady singing, usually concrete evidence that death had occurred.

I prepared to pay my last respects to my old friend. Although I have no religious beliefs, when a patient of mine dies I like to touch their hands one last time, a final salute, a recognition of the end of our shared journey, but my sober mien was disturbed when, on entering his room, I found, not a coffin and a corpse, but a bed and a very-much-alive patient.

I could tell he wasn't dead; he looked too sick and old, the undertaker hadn't had a chance to touch him up yet.

I'll not pretend he was chirpy or singing along, but there was no sign that the hubbub was distressing him.

His wife explained helplessly that the wake had not been planned, but had just … happened; one or two neighbours had heard a rumour and drifted in, then one or two more had seen *them* drifting in, and soon the rush had become unstoppable. This was not a sign of malign intent; it's just what neighbours *do* in Ireland, especially if the local Gaelic football team aren't playing.

Using the full authority of my ancient profession, I shushed the crowd, smashed the fiddle, poured the whiskey down the sink, and stuffed a cream bun in the fat lady's mouth, allowing my friend a few quiet moments alone with his family. When I returned to the kitchen a few minutes later a respectful silence still prevailed.

'How is he, Doctor?' inquired a voice from the back.

'You thought it was all over,' I said, the words rising unbidden, 'It is—now.'

Words failed me

BMJ 23 October 1999

When you English first came to Ireland you despoiled our relics, cut down all our ancient trees, pillaged our women, and made rude noises at our menfolk. But we got the better of you; we loved every second of it, and as a bonus we got the English language, the heritage of Shakespeare and Milton, with all its capacity for bombast and subtlety, pageantry and nuance, a star-crossed marriage of a people gifted with a wild imagination with a vehicle sufficiently complex and idiosyncratic to allow them expression.

Even so, the vagaries of general practice can yet leave us lost for words; the skill of extemporaneous dissembling is not taught in the textbooks.

'I'm bucked, Doctor,' said Jimmy from his sick bed.

'Don't worry, man,' I said, faking a heavy Jamaican accent in a despairing attempt at humour, caught as I was between the Scylla and Charybdis of trying to reassure him without actually telling him lies. 'The fluid tablets will help your breathing and the antibiotics will take care of the chest infection; you'll feel much better in the morning, and I'll see you then.'

I went outside to find the whole family assembled.

'How is he, doctor?' asked his wife anxiously.

I paused, aware that they were hanging on my every word. I was also aware that words are inadequate here. Even the English language in all its meandering glory and richness of texture cannot quite seem to convey that there is a sick old man in there. I'm sure he's dying, body falling apart, all systems are failing, heart, lung, kidneys, brain, you name it.

Although I'm doing my best to keep him comfortable I don't really know what's going on, perhaps only that doing nothing heroic is the right thing; don't really know what's wrong with him; pay no attention to what I write on the death certificate, only guessing; and most of all I don't know how to explain my sense of uncertainty and inadequacy to you because I know it's not what you want to hear right now. You want someone strong and certain and positive, someone who knows what is happening, someone in control.

So: 'Mary,' I said gravely, placing a firm, supportive hand on her shoulder, in the hope that my body language might help disguise the poverty of my words, 'I'm afraid he's bucked.'

Go gently, please

BMJ 6 August 2002

One of our most solemn duties is to confirm that life has fled away into the darkness and can no longer claim any pension entitlements. Sometimes this can be easy, like when there's no head, but sometimes it can be a tough call, and once I got it very wrong.

I had known Jimmy many years ago, so when I saw his widow I went over to pay my respects. I was embarrassed that I hadn't attended the wake, so I over-compensated a bit. I talked about how much I missed Jimmy and what great friends we'd been and all the divilment we used to get up to. The widow seemed rather cool, which I presumed was because of my non-appearance at the wake, so, digging myself deeper, I became even more frenzied in my protestations.

Then, in the middle of an apocryphal story about tying a sheep to a racing car, who should I see coming up the road but Jimmy himself, very much alive. Fortunately, I hadn't yet used any definitive phrases to denote that I thought he was actually dead, such as 'I heard it was a gigantic funeral,' but at this stage the horses were running away with me, and I found myself helplessly continuing the charade.

'Jimmy,' I cried, running up and giving him a comradely pummelling and a big hug. Jimmy was palpably mystified, but we men are simple creatures and my false bonhomie was infectious and irresistible; he gamely responded, and we performed a joyous little *pas de deux* in the middle of the street while the townsfolk gazed on in wild and bewildered surmise.

But we learn from our mistakes.

Dorothy Parker was holding court in the Algonquin Round Table when she heard the news that former US president Calvin Coolidge was dead.

'Really?' she said, 'How can they tell?'

Her cruel little *bon mot* was closer to the truth than she realised; it can be damn hard to tell. If the head is half-hanging off, of course, it's easy, but often life doesn't end at a clear and obvious discrete moment. Sometimes it fades, like a summer night falling, gradually, slowly, softly, easily. The body just does not suddenly shut down and stop; like a car being switched off, parts of it remain warm for a while, and some of the cogs and wheels may continue to turn. The muscles may give one last twitch, the bowels one last playful gurgle, the chest one last heave, the pelvis one last suggestive thrust.

So at what point exactly has death occurred and the spirit left the body? In hospital there are plenty of electronic gizmos, objective ways of confirming death, as well as plenty of second opinions available. But out in the sticks a doctor has to rely on the traditional signs to make a correct diagnosis; no heartbeat, fixed and dilated pupils, absence of breath sounds, shunting in the retinal blood vessels (don't we all check for this; no, seriously).

Make the call, trust your judgement, and ignore the funny noises coming from the death-bed. It's an archetypal example of performative utterance; we're dead because the doc says we are.

All doctors have been in that kitchen, dispensing tea and sympathy, when a relative rushes in; 'Granny's still breathing,' is the accusing shout.

Now is the time to hold your nerve, look them steadily in the eyes, take another scone (freshly baked is traditional), and give the old lady time and space to comply with your diagnosis; breathing space, so to speak (maybe sneak back in later with a pastry-fork, just to be sure, and to tie her shoelaces together in case she becomes a zombie).

Nonetheless, at my funeral, just before they bury me beneath the old sod alongside my fathers and forefathers, could somebody please scratch my eyeballs with a pastry-fork?

Good career move

GP 17 January 2014

I don't usually attend funerals - I've experienced too many accusing looks from the cortege and there's always some bright spark who will shout: 'Why didn't you send him for an X-ray?' or, 'You should have given him an antibiotic.'

But when Father Joe is presiding, I make an exception, in the expectation of what we locals call 'a bit o' diversion'.

'Paddy was a great traveller,' Father Joe once said, 'so it is fitting that his last journey was the one before he died.' Very Zen, leaving the congregation scratching their heads in confusion.

He could also be entertainingly inaccurate.

'Mary-Kate was an angel,' he said. 'Throughout her long illness, she never complained once.'

There was a stifled snigger and some knowing smirks from the pews, and Mary-Kate's relatives smiled wanly at one another.

He, of course, was oblivious to this undercurrent; on his visits, Mary-Kate was all sweetness and light, as the persecuted family members served tea and freshly-baked scones.

The truth was that Mary-Kate spent her declining years gleefully tormenting her nearest and dearest. This, unfortunately, included me, because I made the mistake of visiting too often and familiarity had bred bitter, enduring contempt; if doctors were drinks, I was three-week-old sour milk with cat hairs in it.

On each visit, Mary-Kate would be sitting beside the fire in voluminous black skirts, assiduously cultivating her erythema ab igne, surrounded by her whey-faced, browbeaten daughters-in-law.

'Oh, it's you,' she'd say dismissively. 'What about an X-ray, my leg is giving me gyp and those tablets you gave me were no good.'

I did have some sympathy for Mary-Kate - being the centre of the universe must be a tough job, so I would sit back and let the familiar litany of complaints wash over me.

But who can comprehend the human heart? When we at last lowered Mary-Kate onto Abraham's unfortunate bosom, I actually heard a few tears being shed.

'Good career move, Mary-Kate,' I thought.

Good news or bad?

Irish Times Sat, Nov 5, 2011

'I thought you were dead.'

Footnote; This is an example of flash fiction i.e. fiction of extreme brevity.

Death, a heavy burden...

GP 28 October 2013

My native village, Rostrevor, in Northern Ireland, is ensconced at the foot of the Mourne mountains. The scenery is stunning, the inspiration for CS Lewis's Narnia or Middle-Earth or whatever (somewhere men dress in tights, essentially), and for the famous lyrics: 'Where the mountains of Mourne sweep down to the sea/Like a short fat lady in a long leather dress'. (OK, I added that last bit myself).

But there is a dark side; to get anywhere there, you have to walk uphill.

We Celts are notorious for the exuberance of our emotions, and the Farrell clan is no exception. So you cry at weddings? That don't amount to a hill of beans. We cry at baptisms, birthdays, Christmas, Easter, St Paddy's Day, during sad songs, or just randomly—we're quite competitive over who starts blubbering first.

And funerals—we yield to none in our unabashed exhibitions of public grief. Distant relatives who haven't seen us for years stand back in amazement as apparently total strangers rend their hair and wail like demented wolverines. If I've had to forcibly restrain one grieving widow from throwing herself into the grave after the coffin I've had to restrain twenty. And, of course, once one does it, everyone has to do it, in case people would think they didn't care.

It used to be easier; after the service, we'd pop the coffin in the hearse and drive up, but a few years ago our cousins insisted on carrying Uncle Paid the whole way from their home to the graveyard. Our ancient graveyard,

345

which predates Christianity, is picturesquely but inconveniently sited at the top of a hill and is one hell of a carry.

Previous accepted practice had been to use the hearse for most of the journey and rely on muscle power for only the last few theatrical yards. But yet again, one family sets a precedent, and the spectacle of corteges pitifully collapsing in exhaustion halfway up the hill has now become common; and if the funeral was small, a shortage of pallbearers was another possibility.

On one occasion, strolling along having a pleasant chat at the back, I was called to take a turn.

'Hey,' I felt like saying, 'I didn't know him well; and I didn't like him much.' But, willy-nilly, I took my place at the rear of the coffin, which turned out to be a tactical error. The pallbearer on the other side was much shorter than me, so all the weight was crushing down on my clavicle. Did I mention it was uphill, raining, the wind was against us and the deceased was a big fat guy?

The pain was excruciating, and I almost put the coffin down and admitted, 'I'm not strong enough, he's too heavy,' but this would have shamed my family and its seed, breed and generation, might as well stand up and admit you are only half a man.

However, I didn't become a doctor by being stupid.

With my free hand, in a clandestine manner, I gradually pushed the coffin sideways, transferring the load on to Shorty's neck. Soon, strangulating noises were audible, and the coffin was listing, ready to topple. The cortege rushed forward in alarm, my burden was relieved, and I gilded the lily by ministering with *faux* concern to Shorty, by now blue in the face.

In medicine, if you can fake sincerity, you've got it made. As a senior colleague once said to me: 'There's nothing worse than a smiling bastard.'

This all sounds like a lot of fun, but there is grave purpose afoot. Stifled grief is unconsoled grief, and getting rid of it in one blaze of glory is undoubtedly therapeutic. I know this is wishful thinking and the funeral is not the final act; grief can never be so easily forgotten.

But life must go on, and consequently the aforesaid grieving widows, having had their catharsis, can take a moment out to freshen up their mascara, shimmy right out of that black dress, and start flirting with the undertaker.

You cannot lower your risk of dying...

24 October 2017

Joe has strong views on death; he's against it.

'I read in the paper,' he said, 'that drinking coffee lowers your risk of dying.'

'Joe,' I said kindly, but with just a hint of malice. 'Even the most vacuous, spurious, and sensationalist newspaper headlines always have a kernel of truth. Except for the times they don't. This report is misleading; you cannot lower your risk of dying. It's not optional, some day you will no longer be around to charm and delight future generations in the many, many ways you have charmed and delighted us.'

Death is simple, but vastly complicated. There is a cognitive dissonance here; we know we are going to die, but we don't really know it. It's down the road a bit, just round the corner, out of sight, and we wouldn't thank anyone for informing us precisely the date of our future demise; we prefer to let ill tidings tell themselves when they be felt.

As we get older, the evidence for our certain demise accumulates; sickness piles on sickness, cancer piles upon degenerative disease, piles pile upon piles. It's a grim prospect, but as usual, cognitive dissonance makes the world go round and stops us all being depressed by our own mortality and the weakness and fragility of our flesh.

And who wants to live forever? As Tennyson said: 'Old men must die, else the earth grow mouldy'; from Tithonus babbling endlessly in loathsome old age in the palace of dawn, to the sad plight of the struldbrugs in Gulliver's Travels, the perils of immortality have been well signposted.

The first man to become immortal (or more strictly speaking amortal, you can always get hit by a bus) will be a hero; they'll fete him and praise him, and he'll definitely get laid. But then jealousy and rancour will set in, and our hero will realise that boredom is the new black.

'Joe, I said, 'You and I shall grow old and diminish together, and share a comfortable and mellow dotage.'

Even speaking these words made me depressed; a dread vista, Joe and I, together, for years and years, …

'Not if Trump starts a nuclear war first,' he said.

'Every cloud has a silver lining,' I said.

Death; the bright side

GP 26 June 2015

Death gets a bad rap, but in the late and much-lamented Terry Pratchett's wonderful Discworld novels, Death is humanised.

Perhaps a bit stereotyped – hooded, skeletal, carries a scythe, speaks in a sepulchral tone – he also struggles with the same doubts and uncertainties as the rest of us. And Death would be even more confused by the conceits of modern medicine.

Life used to be so simple – you're born, you live, you die. But it's more complicated now – it's more like you're born, you live, you die, you get CPR, you may or may not die, or end up with a few broken ribs and some hypoxic brain injury just for show, you tweet about it, then you die again, and get CPR again, this time you're really dead, probably exhausted and with a certain sense of relief. Death, where is thy sting?

Terry Pratchett's Death would be getting restless, having to hang around for 10-20 minutes twiddling his bony fingers. 'Give the poor guy a break, I've got other people to see,' he'd be saying.

CPR has become the default treatment for everyone who dies; unless we explicitly forbid it, we will all leave this world the same way. No-one is allowed to die peacefully anymore; instead we'll have someone pounding on our chest, tubes rammed down our throat, multiple needle jabs, our shirts ripped off and electric shocks administered, and all of it a very public spectacle, as an audience has become traditional.

CPR was introduced in 1960, when a team at Johns Hopkins University in Baltimore, Maryland, US, reported its experience with 20 patients on whom they used a new technique, closed-chest cardiac massage. CPR has been a tremendous advance, helped significantly by being so media-friendly; what could be more praiseworthy and melodramatic than resurrecting the dead?

Medical soaps just love CPR, although their success rates are totally unrealistic. Also unrealistic are their patients; usually young, attractive, TV-friendly victims, who have suffered some common, everyday incident like a lightning strike. In reality, most CPR is performed on older patients, with a success rate of zero to 18%.

CPR is not risk-free; it can lead to prolonged suffering, neurological damage and an undignified demise. When our time's up, we should depart gracefully, hopefully leaving a lot of bad debts for future generations to worry about; after all, what have future generations ever done for us?

Death may be the end of the journey, but what really matters is the journey. It's not a defeat, but viewing it as a defeat leads to some of the worst excesses and abuses of modern medicine. This isn't solely our fault; pressure from well-meaning relatives and the inertia of medical bureaucracy only serve to paralyse our attempts to do our best for our patients.

But we should take back that duty, make a stand. The buck stops with us and legal niceties shouldn't prevent us from making the call in our patient's best interests.

Death is an uncomfortable subject, but encouraging patients to investigate and sign an advance care directive would strengthen our hand. And it would be better to do it while they are still healthy, so we're not seen as attempting to hasten the transition to the choir invisible.

Next week: Satan, not such a bad chap.

Chapter 15

Medical Maxims

La Rochefoucauld, a 17th-century philosopher who thought all behaviour was determined by what he called 'self love', distilled his beliefs into a number of maxims. Penguin Classics used to produce a nice edition and at college always I carried a copy around, to appeal to the more intellectual girls.

In homage to the great man, after 30 years in practice, I have developed a few maxims of my own, the medical equivalent of not invading Russia during the winter and never playing dice with a Sicilian when death is on the line: most are particularly addressed to young doctors, and previously shared on twitter, with the hashtag #TipsForNewDocs.

I must also tip my hat to the wonderful Dr Mark Reid, whose 'Medical axioms' has a whole bookful of similar wisdom.

- Drinking three litres of laxative before having a colonoscopy is an ordeal every doctor should endure before inflicting it on others.

- There is, in the misfortune of other doctors, something not entirely unpleasant.

- Doctors should never wear suede shoes.

- On a home visit, if all the furniture is thrashed but the TV and Sky Box remain intact, there is no psychosis involved.

- It is easier to be wise for our patients than for ourselves.

- The more I see of patients, the more I like my dog (adapted from Mark Twain).

- There are lies, damned lies and statistics, and then there are the graphs that drug reps show you (also adapted from Mark Twain).

- Not everything that can be counted counts and not everything that counts can be counted.

- Demand to cut bureaucracy leads to conferences, workshops and training courses on how to cut bureaucracy.

- No drug has yet been invented that will make you good-looking and popular with the opposite sex.

- You can learn something new every day, even from drug reps - for example, never marinate yourself in cologne overnight.

- The light at the end of the tunnel means you are having a colonoscopy, and what's worse, you're awake.

- In any photo of any medical meeting, the good-looking ones are always the drug reps.

- Never condone medical mistakes. Except when you make them, of course.

- Sometimes someone will have to do something, and you'll be the only one who can do anything.

- Don't appeared naked in a fundraising calendar; we know fundraising is a handy excuse, you just like getting your kit off.

- The hardest part of medicine is knowing when not to use it.

- Sometimes there's no right thing to do, just the least wrong thing; that's real medicine for you.

- When I was a lad, undermining other junior docs was an essential ingredient of career progression; what fun we had.

- In medicine, what's right and what's necessary aren't always the same thing.

- Being a patient, like being homeless, is a full-time, 24/7, exhausting job.

- Osler advised equanimity as the second most important medical virtue, next to sarcasm, of course.

- Patients can be bastards, just like everyone else.

- When the Zombie Apocalypse occurs, when anyone dies, tie their shoelaces together. Hilarity will ensuc!!

- Shaking hands is now considered unhygienic, twerking a safer method of greeting patients. It's etiquette for doctors to go first.

- Your patient will have been waiting for you, sometimes for hours/weeks/months, so no matter how busy you are, give them your full attention.

- Be a whistleblower; go on, wreck your career.

- Be strong in will; to strive, to seek, to find, + not to yield, especially to insalubrious body fluids.

- On home visits, if the guard-dog has three heads, you're in big trouble.

- Just because all the clinical findings and tests are normal, doesn't mean there's nothing wrong.

- Context is crucial; called to the 'hood, with pimps jumping on the bonnet, a croquet injury is unlikely.

- Doctors are the natural attorneys of the poor; never lose the rage to effect change.

- A truly ill person will not come up with incredible sound effects.

- Someone rolling around in pain is not in real pain (with some exceptions)

- Touch your patients; there is primal reassurance in being touched, knowing someone close wants to touch you.

- Patients like to inspect the results of an ear syringe and will be disappointed if they don't see big stuff.

- In medicine, there is always somebody out to get you.

- You can do nothing without a form, but there is a form for everything, including ordering more forms.

- If you haven't filled out a form, what you've done hasn't actually happened.

- Always sit the drug rep on a plastic seat that makes amusing farting noises whenever they shift position. Then pointedly open a window.

- When shaking hands with a drug rep, smear some lubricant on your hand first, just for a laugh.

- The more clothes to be removed, the less likely any relevant clinical finding.

- Often what a patient needs most is a warm bath, a hot meal, a soft bed, some kindness, and the gentle touch of a human hand.

- When body fluids are splashing around freely they will inevitably choose the most awkward destination.

- Confusion is not an ignoble state, while certainty is a ridiculous one.

- Don't address patients by their first names.

- Be understanding of human frailty because you also are human and frail.

- Always ask the carer, 'How are you?'

- Look out for immigrants and treat them like you'd want our own exiles to be treated.

- I learnt as much about the human mind from Dostoyevsky's *Crime and Punishment* as from any psychiatry textbook.

- There may be nothing wrong with your patient, but sometimes Nothing Can Be A Real Cool Hand.

- Doughnuts are important.

- Medicine is a cesspool of greedy doctors and whiny patients; there is also a negative side.

- As with a tip for the horses, the responsibility for advice lies not with the donor but with the recipient.

- The skill of extemporaneous dissembling, like most practical skills, is not taught in the textbooks.

- Hunters: 'Never get between a she-bear + her cubs.' Docs; 'Never get between an elderly lady + her tablets.'

- You know it, we all know it: a doctor's most secret and unholy joy is making another doctor look like a klutz.

- When writing sick notes, 'asthenia' sounds more plausible than just 'pure lazy.'.

- Once you become a doctor, everyone else in the world automatically falls into the category 'patient.'

- When you look annoyed all the time, people will think you're busy and ask someone else.

- If trouble erupts in A&E, be ready to fling yourself heroically behind a desk or grab a human shield. A baby is traditional.

- A drab delivering in a ditch, or some dull opiate being emptied to the drains; whatever it is, we have to handle it.

- No-one should be so sick/vulnerable/afraid/alone that we won't be there, reaching out a hand to cure or comfort.

- Always carry a biro in case you get a chance to perform an emergency tracheostomy and Meg Ryan will then sleep with you.

- In medicine there's always a choice. The options might really suck, but doesn't mean there isn't a choice.

- We don't strive to give patients what they want, but what they need.

- Patients aren't your buddies; their expectations and their best interests often conflict.

- If you hear hoofbeats, it's probably not a zebra (unless you're practicing in the Serengeti).

- It's a great privilege to be able to be good to people.

- People are multi-dimensional; 'patient' is only one dimension.

- Every specialist fondly believes, in their hearts, that their specialty is the most important one.

- When attacked by zombies, decapitation is the treatment of choice.

- Always do the unexpected; never let the enemy know what you are thinking.

- It is our vocation to care for everybody, no matter how needy or deluded or repulsive.

- Drug reps are very friendly; they are paid to be your friend.

- Over the years cultivate a tranquil demeanour, which the casual observer might misinterpret as apathy.

- Introduce yourself as a doctor at an emergency, and everyone else will immediately think, 'great, it's not my problem anymore.'

- Dissimulation is a skill every doctor must learn to blithely apply.

- There's no such thing as someone who's well, just someone who hasn't been investigated enough.

- If you can fake empathy, you've got it made.

- A symptom's absence may sometimes be as telling as its presence.

- To speed up a clinic, hide the patient's chair behind the sharps box, so if they do try to sit down, they risk a nasty prick.

- The doctor-patient relationship should not include inadvertently sharing body fluids.

- How to cheer up patients; 'You're not chronically ill, you're medically interesting.'

- Often the best thing to do is let the hare sit.

- Avoid the annual Christmas party for the elderly, which usually turns into a vodka-fueled orgy of gargantuan proportions.

- Sometimes all we can do is listen.

- Confirming death can be easy, like when there's no head, but sometimes can be a tough call. Trust your judgment, and ignore funny noises coming from the death-bed.

- Forget bacteria, trauma, auto-immunity etc, what really screws up people is relationships.

- If you have nothing to say, say it.

- Be a lover, not a fighter.

- To paraphrase the Fat Man; in any emergency, the first thing to do is take your own pulse.

- On home visits, always wear a stethoscope, so you won't be mistaken for the TV licence man.

- If your patient is convulsing, but still tweeting or texting, diagnose a pseudoseizure.

And above all; be kind. It can't be seen or touched or counted, but it's very real; many important things are like that.

And Finally...

When the day of judgment arrives

GP 25 April 2017

When we die, after having CPR and a few complimentary broken ribs, religious folk believe that we present ourselves at the Gates of Heaven, there to be judged on whether we were naughty or nice.

It would seem more efficient if patients provided their medical records at that time; though not a indicator of morality or lack of (there are many more aspects to patients than just being patients), they are a womb-to-tomb record, from which St Peter might make appropriate inferences.

In Joe's case, when he turns up with his records in a celestial wheelbarrow, St Peter will say, 'I don't know about you yet, Joe, but your doctor had a saint's patience.'

Pick your patients more carefully than your friends, I say, because your patients will be with you longer. 'Of all that is written, I love only what a person hath written with his blood,' said Nietzsche. He would have simply adored Joe's medical records, which have been laced with my blood, spiced with a generous helping of sweat and the occasional tear as well, in fact every possible body fluid except semen. They could be read in a fortnight or two (or three), if that was your idea of a good time.

When I retired, I realised I was handing over Joe's case to another doctor. If I'd wanted to be really helpful, I could have put a (removable) sticky on the front of that fat file; 'Ignore everything inside,' it might have said. The case summary would read, 'Joe always thinks he is sick, but is always well; just keep telling him what he doesn't have; any really important things in here are drowned in a sea of irrelevance.'

But then I remembered all the dark days, and how my heart would sink when that huge set of notes (and that was volume six only) would come thumping down on the desk in front of me (I'd feel oddly disappointed that the desk didn't actually collapse) as Joe sat down and engineered one chubby knee over the other.

'Just let me go outside to cry for a moment,' I'd say to him. Joe's multitudinous complaints were reliable and consistent, and even, in an ever-more rapidly changing world, sort of comforting. Only not very.

I'd suffered, and now, at last, it was someone else's turn.

One last look back…

GP 12 May 2017

On the day I retired from practice I remember standing at the door looking back at my surgery one last time.

The room where I had spent so many years of my life, where I had fought the long defeat, always believing that I could make things better for someone else, if not always for myself.

And over those years I'd made some tragic mistakes, understandable in retrospect, but reason and guilt don't speak the same language, for there is sorrow baked into the clay and stone of which the world is made.

I'd learned some painful lessons, but in life the things that are good for you in the long run hurt for a little while when you first get to them.

The tatty diplomas on the walls, the chair moulded into the shape of my buttocks; so many memories, some good, some bad, some amusing, some mildly nauseating, there are a million stories in the naked surgery. It was more than just a room, it was a crucible, bearing witness to all, from the worried well to the first cold intimations of mortality.

There, tucked away in the corner, the canary-yellow sharp's box in which little Charley somehow contrived to get his head stuck (we could tell he was stuck by his screams); how we laughed.

'Should we get him out?' said his mother.

'Only if you want him to live,' I said. 'Otherwise it's optional.'

And, there on the wall, just the slightest smudge on the soothing vomit-green paint, evidence of the time Joe's sebaceous cyst exploded as he poked at it. This was not a positive development, pungent caseous material cascading all over the room. It hit the walls and ceiling, the computer, the desk, and, in accordance with the universal rules of humour, my Ralph Lauren shirt; it smelt as if a cat had died for weeks afterward, and patients would occasionally faint (so it wasn't all in vain).

'For feck's sake, Joe,' I said.

'I'm sorry,' he said, always ready with the repartee, 'I wasn't aware there was a protocol.'

I was either happy to leave or sad to go, and one of these was more likely than the other.

'Let's get out of here,' I said to myself.

'Agreed,' I replied.

The rest is silence.

CPSIA information can be obtained
at www.ICGtesting.com
Printed in the USA
LVHW021135160619
621371LV00003B/665